# DRUGS, SPORT, AND POLITICS

**Robert Voy, MD**
with Kirk D. Deeter

**Leisure Press**
Champaign, Illinois

**Library of Congress Cataloging-in-Publication Data**

Voy, Robert O., 1933-
  Drugs, sport, and politics / by Robert Voy.
    p. cm.
  ISBN 0-88011-409-6
  1. Doping in sports.  2. Doping in sports--Political aspects.
  I. Title.
  RC1230.V68  1991
  362.29'08'8796--dc20                                      90-38241
                                                               CIP

ISBN: 0-88011-409-6

Acquisitions Editor: Brian Holding
Developmental Editor: Holly Gilly
Assistant Editors: Dawn Levy, Julia Anderson
Copyeditor: Peter Nelson
Proofreader: Pam Johnson
Indexer: Sheila Ary
Production Director: Ernie Noa
Typesetters: Sandra Meier, Angela K. Snyder, Brad Colson
Text Design: Keith Blomberg
Text Layout: Tara Welsch
Cover Design: Jack Davis
Cover Photo: Wilmer Zehr
Interior Art: Denise Lowry
Printer: Braun-Brumfield, Inc.

Printed in the United States of America

10  9  8  7  6  5  4  3  2  1

**Leisure Press**
A Division of Human Kinetics Publishers, Inc.
Box 5076, Champaign, IL 61825-5076
1-800-747-4457

*U.K. Office:*
**Human Kinetics Publishers (UK) Ltd.**
PO Box 18
Rawdon, Leeds LS19 6TG
England
(0532) 504211

For my family,
and the many athletes who keep the Olympic dream alive.

# Contents

## Prescription for Reform

# Acknowledgments

My sincere appreciation goes out to these individuals and groups:

- My family, Ann, Kim, Bill, and Dan, for their support throughout.
- William Simon and Col. F. Don Miller for giving me an opportunity to serve the United States Olympic Committee. Special acknowledgment to Col. Miller for his ever-present leadership training and advice.
- Gen. George Miller, who I still believe is the best man to run the USOC.
- Baaron B. Pittenger, Kenneth "Casey" Clarke, PhD, and Georgia McDonald, who taught me about sports administration.
- Lajuan Conner and Ernie Hinck, now with the United States Olympic Foundation. They showed me the ropes of protocol and finance.
- Sheryl Abbot, director of the Olympic job opportunities program, for her vision of what our athletes need to continue their Olympic dreams.
- Ronald T. Rowan, general counsel, who was always available to lend advice and a pail to help bail me out when the water rose in the boat.
- Linda Burke, director of human resources, who taught me that employees who are treated appropriately will work appropriately, loyally, and efficiently.
- Frank Aires, international games preparation and logistics coordinator, who almost single-handedly put our athletes on the playing field, clothed and equipped, from Colorado Springs to Sarajevo, Yugoslavia.
- Theresa Dolezal, tour coordinator, and the guides like Jackie Murray, who put the Olympic Training Center's best foot forward to visitors.
- Sheila M. Walker, director of Olympic Festivals and Competitions, who is, in my estimation, the best sports event coordinator in the U.S. She always remembered the second cousins—drug control crews—at the Festivals.

- Larry McCollum, director of the Olympic Training Centers, a former marine, a superb administrator, and a leader in probably the toughest job in the U.S. Olympic organization.
- Marguerite Gigliello, assistant director of the Training Center, who always knew the best way to handle the athletes' personal and social problems.
- Kevin Moody and the struggling sports medicine staffs at Lake Placid, New York, and Marquette, Michigan, who managed the Outreach sports medicine program while given nothing more than promises that as yet haven't been fulfilled.
- Art Brandt, a veteran manager of the sports center and a continuous provider of space and opportunity for sport activity, day or night.
- Sweela Hortick, Ivette Hernandez, Lavon Venard, and the others at the USOC–United Airlines travel office.
- Mike Moran, USOC director of public information and media relations, and his staff, Bob Condron and Gayle Plant, who realized the value of the Division of Sports Medicine and Science's direct services to athletes and worked overtime to report our successes. They understand!
- Marv Perham and Joe Laurie for their knowledge and unique way of providing security and safety on the campus.
- The buildings and grounds staff, particularly Rick Miner, who were always there through rain, hail, and snowstorms.
- Jeanette Grice, my loyal administrative assistant and troubleshooter, for her knowledge of protocol, budget, and organizational skills. I could not have made it without her.
- My dedicated staff of over 40 persons, who constituted the Division of Sports Medicine and Science; personal friend, colleague, and former director Chuck Dillman, PhD; Sarah Smith, PhD, who stuck in there when we needed her; Peter Van Handel, PhD, who just did the work and let the politics go by; and the computer genius of those such as Leonard Jansen. Sports Science maintained its base throughout storms of criticism and organizational doubts of its effectiveness.
- Bob Beeten, Jenny Stone, and the athletic training staff, who taught me the importance of the coach and the trainer.
- Ann Grandjean, EdD, RD, director of the International Center for Sports Nutrition in Omaha, Nebraska, for bringing nutrition to a new level of importance in sport.
- My personal staff: Rose, Joanie, Mary, Renee, Helen, Cindy, Eddie, and Buddy. It was sometimes the worst of times, but we all made it the best of times together.
- Don Catlin, MD, and Caroline Hatton, PhD, for their thankless efforts behind the drug program scene to crank out testing results in an irrefutable manner, and for the scientific resources they provided, which made the USOC drug control program the model for the world.

- The many volunteer physicians who served as my "board of directors," some on the Sports Medicine Council, the Drug Control Committee, and the Exercise-Induced Bronchospasm Project—to name a few, Irv Dardik, MD, Bob Leach, MD, Bert Zarins, MD, Roy Bergman, MD, Dan Hanley, MD, Jim Puffer, MD, Jack Wilmore, PhD, Jerry May, PhD, Bill Pierson, MD, James Betts, MD—and over 150 volunteer physicians and athletic trainers throughout the country.
- The many who think as I do on these issues but don't necessarily speak up or speak out on the subject. I feel I left behind many, many kindred spirits, who I hope will take up the lead for creative change.
- All the friends and sport federation personnel who worked cooperatively with Sports Medicine and Science to effect some of the changes and programs suggested in this book.
- The 30 loyal drug-testing crew chiefs, who made the USOC drug control program so successful.
- The Johnson & Johnson Company, which deserves special appreciation for its in-kind annual supply of all the medical and health equipment we needed at the United States Olympic Training Center.
- The private foundations that gave tens of thousands of dollars in equipment and asked for no recognition in return. They made the difference and kept my program state of the art.
- Judy Nelson and Dr. Hildebrand for providing superior athlete dental care.
- Thomas Mahony, MD, my chief orthopedic consultant and coordinator of medical services in the Colorado Springs medical community.
- Bruce Wilhelm, a friend and confidant.

R. Voy

# *Additional Acknowledgments*

Thanks to

- Ira Josephs, a good friend and a gifted sportswriter, whose assistance was a tremendous asset to this project.
- Sports editor Jay Nagle of the *Intelligencer* in Doylestown, Pennsylvania, for his patience and flexibility.
- Bob Voy, who began this project as a partner and finished it as a friend.

K. Deeter

# Introduction

The United States Olympic movement is facing some serious crises. I believe that in many ways, unfortunately, the United States Olympic Committee and various sport national governing bodies are ill-equipped to meet these challenges.

The use of performance enhancing drugs by Olympic athletes has only recently become a public issue, though it has been a serious problem in the sports community for many years. Some sports officials have begun to address this crisis and initiate programs to bring about change; however, I believe we still have a long, long way to go before the situation will ever be fully resolved.

When Canadian sprinter Ben Johnson tested positive for using the anabolic-androgenic steroid (AAS) stanozolol after he won the gold medal and broke his own world record with a time of 9.79 seconds in the men's 100-meter dash at the 1988 Olympic Games in Seoul, the world of sport was sent reeling from the blow to its image. Sports fans around the globe felt betrayed. For some, this was their introduction to the uglier side of the Olympic Games.

I'm here to say that the use of anabolic-androgenic steroids and other performance enhancing substances has been commonplace in elite-level amateur and professional sports for years. According to many athletes I've worked with, the only thing that separated Johnson from a great number of others who competed in Seoul in a vast variety of sports is simple: He got caught.

In early 1984 I was lured by the opportunity to actually be a part of the Olympic dream, to become the chief medical officer of the United States Olympic Committee (USOC). I had to leave my successful private family medical practice in Tualatin, Oregon, though I realized the move would mean a two-thirds cut in salary and a transition to a new community for my wife, Ann, and me.

But the chance to be in the inner circle of the U.S. Olympic effort, in the position of one of the leading sports medicine authorities in the world, certainly seemed to justify the change. I wanted to serve on the front lines of the American Olympic movement. Because I thought my expertise in the science of sports medicine could help young individuals achieve their highest goals, I approached my new position with charged enthusiasm, excited by the feeling that I had truly "arrived" on the scene of amateur sports and confident that my time at the USOC would be the experience of a lifetime.

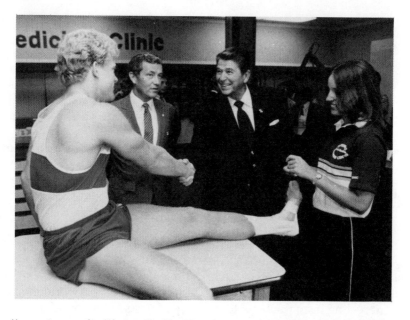

An "experience of a lifetime"—Dr. Voy escorting President Ronald Reagan on a tour of the Sports Medicine Clinic in Colorado Springs.

Indeed, I do feel that during the 5 years I spent in Colorado Springs, I helped U.S. amateur sports programs take significant strides forward in the areas of sports medicine and science. My department improved the technological resources available to help athletes develop rehabilitation programs to recover from injuries. We increased our understanding of the roles diet and nutrition play in athletic performance. We helped coaches and athletes formulate more efficient training regimens. We significantly improved the technology used to test athletes for banned substances. And, through the establishment of a drug hotline, we were able to build a stronger dialogue among coaches, athletes, and the USOC regarding substances banned by the International Olympic Committee

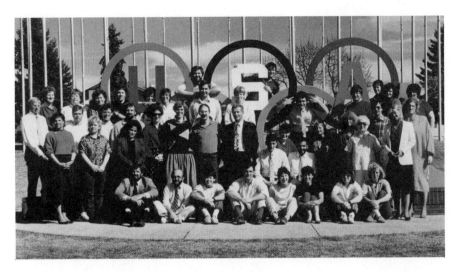

Dr. Voy (in the second row under the *S*) and his Sports Medicine and Science staff at the U.S. Olympic Training Center.

(IOC). In short, I think I helped make the USOC a more reliable scientific resource center for this nation's amateur athletes.

I also enjoyed meeting many talented young individuals, traveling the world, and witnessing the new chapters of Olympic history unfold before my very eyes.

Despite these triumphs, working with the USOC was not always a physician's dream. I discovered the darker, uglier side of the Olympic experience, which has only recently been revealed to the general public, a side tainted by politics, big money, and drugs.

There are probably gold medal winners and world record holders from the United States who would never have even come near the winner's podium had it not been for their use of performance enhancing substances—and this is still happening. What's worse, I also know, after working elbow-to-elbow with elite-level athletes, that many drug users do not *want* to use drugs but feel they *have* to to stay even with everyone else.

This is tragic. Drug use among athletes is probably the most serious threat to the Olympic ideal today. It signifies a great departure from the original purpose of the modern Olympiad. Instead of being a competition and celebration for the body human, the Olympics have in some ways become a mere proving ground for scientists, chemists, and unethical physicians. In my opinion, despite renewed concern about drug use in sports, the Olympic ideal will never fully recover from the impact of this problem until it is absolutely, verifiably eliminated.

My position on drug use in sport is simple: I am vehemently opposed to the use of performance enhancing drugs in any sport at any time.

I base this position on two reasons. First, as a sports enthusiast, I recognize using performance enhancing drugs as cheating, plain and simple. A world record means nothing to me when I know chemical substances played a significant role in that achievement. I'm sick of watching athletes cheat their way onto the winner's podium at the Olympic Games. Moreover, I'm tired of seeing clean athletes, who sacrifice so much to earn a shot at the gold, fall short because they aren't using drugs to enhance their performances. I'd like to see the playing field made level once again. Restoring a level playing field would mean either that all athletes should be allowed to use these drugs legally or that all drug use should be stopped and controlled by strict precompetition and postcompetition testing programs.

Because I am a physician and realize the dangers inherent in drug use, allowing athletes to use performance-enhancing substances is, in my mind, an irresponsible and completely unacceptable approach to creating a level playing field. This physician's perspective is the second reason I oppose drug use in sport.

The medical profession is now beginning to understand that anabolic-androgenic steroids have serious, in some cases lethal, side effects. We now know that by using anabolic-androgenic steroids, a male athlete exposes himself to many risks, including contracting arterial sclerosis, high blood pressure, heart disease, liver cancer, prostate cancer, sterility, and psychological alterations. With the female athlete, anabolic-androgenic steroid use may mean liver cancer, menstrual irregularity, hypertension, depression, and irreversible masculinizing changes such as a deepened voice and even abnormal genitalia.

Despite our warnings, athletes have stuck to their use of performance enhancing drugs—so religiously, in fact, that today anabolic-androgenic steroid sales on the black market are estimated to be a $200 million business.

After talking to athletes and watching this problem fester firsthand for the last several years, I realized the competitors are not to be blamed completely. When one understands that Ben Johnson stood to earn an estimated $30 million in endorsements, appearance fees, and so on had he not been caught, how can he be condemned for taking anabolic-androgenic steroids, especially when he knew a considerable percentage of his competitors were using them as well?

Clearly, the responsibility for correcting the drug problem should rest with the sport governing bodies, which are at this time unable to contain the situation and, through their own ineffectiveness, are allowing an unfair double standard to exist in amateur sports.

While I was still at the USOC, I began to campaign for increased testing, research, and educational resources to combat the problem of drug abuse by athletes. Believe it or not, for all intents and purposes, my pleas fell on deaf ears. In fact, my drug testing budget for the 1989-1992 quadrennium was decreased proportionately from the budget I operated with before the 1988 Games, despite the renewed public concern on the issue.

When I asked USOC President Robert Helmick to explain this decision, the response I got was, ''The USOC can't be all things to all people with regard to the drug issue.'' Reading between the lines, I understood that to mean many people at the USOC were in their business for one reason: to bring home the gold. Just *how* the athletes accomplished that—well, few really cared.

Soon I realized I would have to take my battle somewhere else if I were going to be heard. I resigned as chief medical officer and director of Sports Medicine and Science of the United States Olympic Committee in March of 1989. I felt I owed it to myself and to the many athletes who are negatively affected by the present unfair system that governs amateur sport.

My intent with this book is not to point fingers, not to spread sour grapes, but to try to let people know the facts. To do this, I'll explain which drugs are used to enhance athletic performance and what the effects of those drugs are on the athletes. I'll relate why this issue is such a serious threat to the sports community and why I believe the United States Olympic Committee is not committing itself to stopping the problem. Finally, I'll give some prescriptions for reform that will present concrete solutions to the widespread drug problem plaguing international athletic competition.

There are too many damaging myths and misconceptions floating around the sports world on this volatile subject. Athletes, parents, coaches, trainers, and sports fans deserve to know the history of these drugs, their effects, and the role they play in sports today. You see, the fight to clean up sport is one we will all have to join.

Though I now work on the periphery of the U.S. Olympic movement, I've committed myself to doing whatever it takes to win this battle because I believe the Olympic ideal is a treasure worth fighting for. Since the inception of the modern Olympic movement in 1892, many Americans have grown up mesmerized by the Olympic flame. The torch, the five rings, the flag, and the competitors themselves have grown to represent the ultimate level of athletic competition.

Perhaps what is most special about the Games is that the Olympic spirit transcends the athletes and coaches on the playing field. The Games bring out the dreamer in all of us, and they bring our world together. We all shed a tear with a young athlete as a gold medal is hung around his neck and his national flag is raised before the world. It is in these brief moments that humans are truly united through the spirit of Olympism. Every 4 years, the magic of the Olympics allows us to escape the worries of our lives and feel fervently proud to be members of a world community united in the pursuit of excellence in sport. Sadly, for many, the drugs and politics that have begun to plague the Games in recent years are causing this magic to fade.

Yet, in my eyes, even though I've been exposed to the darker, uglier side of the Games, the Olympic torch has not gone out. I still believe in the Olympic ideal, and I'm still inspired by the majority of athletes who compete clean and reach the top. To them I say: Persevere; we can bring about change together. For them I am writing this book.

I hope this newer, nobler, challenge can help rekindle the flame so that it will once again shine for all the world as a symbol of fairness and honor.

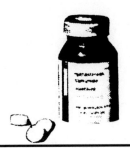

# The Doping
# Game

# 1

## Glory Years

### A Brief History of Doping in Sport

From the ancient fields of Olympus to the modern athletic arenas around the globe, sports competitions have fueled the fire of people's instinctive quest for excellence. Sport is a vehicle that allows the human mind to dream. It has been a source of heroics and inspiration. Throughout the ages, sport has facilitated our struggle to reach higher plateaus and achieve the ultimate thrill of victory.

Sport has also been, to those select few athletes who reach true excellence, an incredible source of spiritual power. To be swifter, stronger, more cunning, or more graceful than the best competition in the world is among the highest aspirations an athlete can have. And to finally reach the pinnacle of success releases a tremendous rush of energy—of personal satisfaction and accomplishment—that few people are ever fortunate enough to experience.

Athletes devote lifetimes of sweat and emotion to the hope of someday tasting this euphoria. In the minds of many athletes, the surge of power that comes with victory is worth virtually any sacrifice. Because of this universal desire to succeed, athletes have forever been searching for a magical route to the winner's podium, some legitimate and others not. Although some athletes have devoted themselves to years of training and personal sacrifice to obtain their ultimate performances, others have sought shortcuts to victory.

I suspect it wasn't too long after the very idea of sport was conceived that athletes learned about the shortcuts to victory, meaning they learned how to cheat. The ancient classic the *Iliad* describes how Odysseus defeated Ajax in a footrace by enlisting the goddess Athena to trip his competitor. Ancient Greek records even indicate the early Olympic Games were tainted by fraud, corruption, and scandal. Indeed, the notion of cheating seems to be as old as sport itself, though today the cheating "goddesses" come in different forms.

There is one type of cheating that has evolved through the ages and is seemingly impossible to gauge and control. It is subtle. It isn't visible to a referee, an umpire, or a judge. The cheating to which I refer happens within the body. Today it is called doping.

Doping, in my mind, is the use of any substance (natural or synthetic) taken into the body by any route—be it by mouth, injected through the skin or into vessels, instilled in the eye or bladder, inhaled into the lungs, or inserted into the rectum—for nontherapeutic reasons to enhance performance. Today sport officials try to control doping with urinalysis testing. This is my area of expertise. Dope testing was one of my main responsibilities while I was working with the United States Olympic Committee (USOC).

When athletes are drug tested, they are asked to produce a urine specimen after they have competed. Using sophisticated technology, we are then able to analyze this sample to find any traces of drugs in the athletes' bodies. Some drugs, like stimulants, are relatively easy to detect because they are short acting and must be taken close in time to the competition to enhance an athlete's performance. Others, however, like anabolic-androgenic steroids, are more difficult to discover because athletes use these drugs at different times of their training cycles to help them build muscle.

Unfortunately, there are numerous ways for athletes to beat the system. I will discuss these subjects in considerable detail a bit later. For now suffice it to say that drug testing just isn't the threat to drug-using athletes one might think it is.

Recently, due to the frenzied media attention on the subject of doping, people have begun to realize just how widespread this form of cheating has become among elite-level athletes, and how many athletes use chemical substances to maximize and enhance performances. The public now knows that athletes, who work so hard to make their bodies strong and healthy, are willing to take serious health risks to gain a competitive edge by using chemical shortcuts. The quest for sports excellence through drug use has given the issue of doping renewed concern among sports officials and the public. In fact, in the past 2 or 3 years alone, steroids and cocaine have become topics of household conversation.

Yet, many people may not realize doping is hardly a new problem to the sports community. In fact, doping has a tradition as long and complicated as sport itself. The average sports enthusiast is staggered when even beginning to understand this incredible history and the tremendous effect doping has had on sport.

Many people understand that anabolic-androgenic steroids (AAS) and stimulants are among some of the categories of drugs used by athletes today. However, I doubt that many sports fans realize AAS and stimulants are just two facets of this complex issue. Human growth hormone (hGH) and blood transfusions are but two of the most recent threats to fairness in sport. Few fans know of the so-called brake drugs being taken by young gymnasts and figure skaters to delay puberty, or the drugs used by shooters to slow their heart rates and minimize the intention tremors of their trigger fingers, enabling these athletes to record expert scores unattainable by natural means.

In my experience, I have encountered very few sports which have not been affected in one way or another by doping.

Doping is defined by the USOC in its 1989-92 drug education handbook as follows:

> According to the International Olympic Committee (IOC), "doping" is the "administration of or use by a competing athlete of any substance foreign to the body or any physiological substance taken in abnormal quantity or taken by an abnormal route of entry into the body with the sole intention of increasing in an artificial and unfair manner his/her performance in competition. When necessity demands medical treatment with any substance which, because of its nature, dosage, or application is able to boost the athlete's performance in competition in an artificial and unfair manner, this too is regarded as doping." To implement the concept, the IOC has derived a list of substances banned for use by athletes in competition, and has developed a drug testing program at the Olympics and related competitions to deter the use of these substances.[1]

The actual word *doping* has an interesting history of its own. Centuries ago, in the native Kaffir dialect of South Africa, *dop* referred to a stimulating liquor used by tribesmen in religious ceremonies. Through assimilation with the language of Afrikaners, the final "e" was added to form the word *dope*. A Dutch form of the word *dop* also surfaced several hundred years ago, yet it wasn't until 1889 that *dop* first appeared in an English dictionary. At that time, dop was defined as a narcotic mixture of opium used for racehorses.

The earliest accounts of doping among human athletes actually go far back to the ancient Olympic Games, whose documents reveal that athletes drank various brandy or wine concoctions or ingested mushrooms to enhance performance.[2] There are even accounts of alkaloids such as strychnine being mixed with alcohol for a stimulant effect. Roman gladiators are said to have taken drugs to enhance performance in the arena, and medieval knights frequently ingested stimulants to prepare them for their jousts. Like modern stimulants, they were used to mask fatigue and pain signals emitted by the central nervous system.

In more recent times, records indicate that in 1865 canal swimmers racing in Amsterdam were charged with taking *dop*, as were a number of cyclists competing throughout Europe. The 6-day cycle racers were using a mixture of heroin and cocaine called speedball to increase endurance. A 6-day cycling event would begin on a given morning and proceed for 144 continuous hours, day and night, before a victor would be declared. During the period when this sport was most popular, Belgian athletes were allegedly taking sugar tablets soaked in ether to create a stimulant effect. To compete with the Belgians, the French athletes were supposedly taking caffeine tablets, and the British were said to be inhaling pure oxygen and taking strychnine, heroin, and cocaine, washed down with brandy—all in attempts to gain some competitive edge.

These cyclists' doping practices caught on like wildfire throughout the world of sport. By the end of the 19th century, prizefighters were also frequently taking alcohol, strychnine, or other concoctions before stepping into the ring.

The first recorded drug-related death in the world of sport occurred in 1886, when an English cyclist died from an overdose of something called trimethyl, which was probably a form of ether.[3]

The doping crisis visibly arrived on the modern Olympic scene during the 1904 Games in St. Louis, when American marathoner Thomas Hicks needed extreme medical measures to be revived after his event because he took large doses of strychnine mixed with raw egg whites during his race. Basically, most of the drugs used in the early modern Olympic Games were a mixture of strychnine and alcohol.

It wasn't until its advent during World War II that amphetamine became the drug of choice over strychnine. Most of us who lived in the 1940s can recall amphetamine's being used frequently by students to study, truck drivers who needed to drive at night, and night-shift factory workers. Amphetamine kept them awake and alert when their bodies needed an added boost to perform.

Given the effectiveness of amphetamine, it wasn't much of a surprise to see it adopted quickly by the athletic community. Some of the first notable amphetamine-related doping cases occurred at the 1952 Olympic Winter Games in Oslo, Norway, where several speed skaters became ill during the preliminary heats and needed medical attention to recover.

Perhaps the landmark amphetamine-related tragedy in Olympic history occurred when Danish cyclist Knud Enemar Jensen collapsed and died during the 175.38-km road race at the 1960 Summer Olympiad in Rome. It was reported at the time that, leading up to his death, Jensen was taking, supposedly on doctor's orders, a combination of nicotynal alcohol and amphetamine, sarcasatically nicknamed by his competitors the "Knud

Jensen diet." Several of the other athletes competing in Jensen's race collapsed like Jensen had at the finish; however, Jensen was the only fatality. An autopsy revealed that Jensen probably died from dehydration by the amphetamine in his system, though his skull had also been fractured.

Another notable death in following years was that of Tommy Simpson of Great Britain, the most acclaimed professional cyclist at that time. Simpson died during the 13th day of the 1967 Tour de France. After he collapsed during the race, a vial of amphetamine was found in his pocket; of course, amphetamine was later discovered in Simpson's body by the pathologist who conducted his autopsy.

---

*Author's Note:* It is interesting to me that professional cyclists have defended their use of stimulants of all types, including amphetamines and caffeine, throughout the years. They have continued to do so even in recent years (see related discussion on Jeannie Longo in chapter 3).

---

In 1968 Yves Mottin died in Grenoble, France, shortly after a cross-country cycling race. Jean-Louis Quadri, a soccer player, died on the playing field, also in Grenoble in 1968. Both deaths were due to amphetamine-related causes.

The casualty list of athletes who died from performance enhancing or "recreational" drug abuse goes on and on. When will it all stop? Despite these tragedies and the lessons they should have taught us, drug use continues to claim the lives of young athletes.

One of the most recent and well-publicized deaths attributed to drug use occurred in 1986. Len Bias, the first-round draft pick of the Boston Celtics, collapsed in his dormitory room on the campus of the University of Maryland after taking cocaine, and died. Bias had the world at his feet. A big NBA contract and professional career awaited him. But one wrong judgment, a sudden impulse, and a deadly drug cost him everything.

Cocaine, generally regarded as the most addicting recreational drug, has become the drug of choice these days among many amateur and professional athletes around the world, both as a recreational drug *and* as a performance enhancing substance.

In his *Sports Illustrated* exposé published March 16, 1987, former Villanova basketball star Gary McLain wrote (p. 49):

> Tuesday, Nov. 17, 1981 marked my first Villanova game, an exhibition against a team from Yugoslavia. I also did my first cocaine that day, in my dormitory room just a few hours before tip-off. . . . I'd heard that guys who did cocaine before games played better. This was already an exciting day. "Yeah," I said. "Let me get some. Let me try a one-and-one" . . . a little spoonful of cocaine up each nostril.[4]

### ATHLETE DRUG-RELATED FATALITY LIST[5]

| Athlete | Sport | Drug | Died |
| --- | --- | --- | --- |
| Dick Howard | Track and field | Amphetamine | 1960 |
| "Big Daddy" Lipscomb | Football | Heroin | 1963 |
| Terry Furlow | Basketball | Cocaine | 1980 |
| Billy Ylvisaker | Polo | Cocaine | 1983 |
| Daniel Baroudi | Bodybuilding | Anabolic-androgenic steroids | 1984 |
| Larry Gordon | Football | Cocaine | 1986 |
| Len Bias | Basketball | Cocaine | 1986 |
| Don Rogers | Football | Cocaine | 1986 |
| Dave Singh | Bodybuilding | Anabolic-androgenic steroids | 1987 |
| Birgit Dressel | Heptathlon | Anabolic-androgenic steroids | 1987 |
| Hernell Jackson | Basketball | Cocaine | 1987 |
| David Croudip | Football | Cocaine | 1988 |
| Rico Marshall | Football | Cocaine | 1988 |

McLain also played in the Wildcats' 1985 Final Four semifinal game against Memphis State high on cocaine. He admitted he would have played high in the final against Georgetown but "didn't have any cocaine available."[6]

As I said before, stimulants are just one facet of this issue. Over 3 decades ago, the athletic community found an equally effective way to chemically enhance performance. These new drugs created power, mass, and endurance. They not only altered the mind, but they actually changed the body. In the late 1950s anabolic-androgenic steroids were thrust onto the sports scene.

It was rumored in the early 1950s that the Soviets had been using hormonal experimentation for some time to help their athletes enhance performances. It was not until the 1956 World Games in Moscow, however, when an American physician, John B. Ziegler, MD (who was a member of the medical staff for the 1956 World Games), actually witnessed the use of anabolic-androgenic steroids (straight testosterone) among

Soviet athletes. It was Dr. Ziegler's insight that actually brought the issue to the surface of sport in the United States for the first time.

In Moscow Ziegler witnessed urinary catheters being used by Soviet athletes. He wasn't surprised by this, because he knew that the use of testosterone would enlarge the prostate gland to the point where the urinary tract would be obstructed, making it difficult for the athletes to urinate. Therefore, the athletes would either catheterize themselves or have their coaches catheterize them so that they would be able to pass their urine. (Several years later, once doping control was instituted in amateur sport, catheterization became a very popular way for athletes to beat drug testing. The athletes would catheterize themselves first to drain their own drug-tainted urine from their bladders, then to pump bogus, "clean" urine into their bodies, which they would pass when tested. This process enabled many athletes to beat the tests; it is still used today by athletes trying to avoid detection.)

Ziegler also noticed that the really good Soviet athletes would be on the scene only during a given competition. They would not be around during the off-season, when withdrawal from anabolic-androgenic steroids would decrease their mammoth muscles. Anyway, in terms of pure performance enhancement, the positive results the Soviets enjoyed in most competitions spoke for themselves.

After the 1956 World Games, Ziegler returned to the United States and began informing the medical and sports communities about the use of anabolic-androgenic steroids by the Soviet athletes. In an attempt to help Western athletes compete more effectively against the Soviets who used testosterone, and in an effort to reduce the bad side effects of testosterone—namely, acne, hair loss, prostate enlargement, and shrinkage of the testicles—Dr. Ziegler aided the CIBA Pharmaceutical Company in the development of Dianabol, or, in generic terms, methandrostenolone. Dianabol, also known as D-bol in the gym, became the American alternative to straight testosterone. It was among the first big-time anabolic-androgenic steroids. Derivatives of Dianabol are still on the market, despite the fact that CIBA has stopped manufacturing it because of the low demand for methandrostenolone in legitimate medical practice.

Dianabol was a derivative of testosterone designed only to create the anabolic (muscle-building) effects of the substance. Ziegler initially planned to extract the radical chemical elements in testosterone that he thought caused the enlargement of the prostate gland and other glands, such as those producing acne. Ziegler thought he could maintain the anabolic effects of testosterone yet decrease the negative side effects that caused discomfort to the athletes. Though he may have succeeded to some extent, we now know even modern-day attempts to rid derivatives of testosterone of the potentially harmful side effects have failed. *To this date no anabolic-androgenic steroid has been developed that causes only muscle growth.*

With the introduction of Dianabol in the late 1950s, anabolic-androgenic steroids really got their initial use. They became popular very rapidly. Athletes were indeed beginning to realize greater strength as a result of using Dianabol, and they were quick to use this newfound advantage during competitions.

They simply couldn't get enough of the stuff. Although the usual therapeutic dose of Dianabol was initially 5 mg one to three times per day, Dr. Ziegler soon found out that athletes were using many times more— sometimes 10 to 20 times more—than the therapeutic dose.

With this discovery, Dr. Ziegler realized the mistake he had made by helping introduce these drugs to the athletic community. It was almost a sports world analogy to the story of Dr. Frankenstein. Soon after Dianabol hit the market, Dr. Ziegler knew he had created a monster, a fact he regretted for the rest of his life.[7]

In Dr. Ziegler's defense, taking pills to enhance performance—any type of performance—was not considered unethical or illegal in the 1950s and 1960s. At that time the general public had just started to accept the notion of polypharmacy. Vitamins had been introduced long before, but they had never received a large amount of popularity. The pharmaceutical industry was introducing many drugs that could be used to benefit health, particularly antibiotics. So physicians began to use prescription drugs more frequently in their practices, and people became more aware that drugs could help them with their maladies. We were a society that was just developing the pill-popping scene. Thus, it was surprising neither that Dr. Ziegler had this interest nor that these drugs became very popular in the athletic community so rapidly. Nevertheless, the era of anabolic-androgenic steroid use was given its humble beginnings.

Bob Goldman, author of the book *Death in the Locker Room* (1984), tells us that "the first notable female athletes who used anabolic-androgenic steroids to gain the competitive edge included European 200-meter dash champion, Maria Itkina of the Soviet Union, Romanian world record high jumper Iolanda Balas, and the Soviet Press sisters—Olympic champion pentathlete Irina Press, and Tamara Press, the 1964 Olympic gold medalist in the shot put and discus events who was also known as 'The Flower of Leningrad.' "[8]

Goldman states: "All four of these women disappeared at high points of their careers after Polish sprinter Ewa Klobukowska ran afoul of the tests following the 1967 European track-and-field championships when her chromosome count cast doubt on her femininity. Anyone taking a look at these 'women' would be hard pressed to remember in them the girl next door (unless you lived next to the New York Jets, of course)."[9]

It has long been assumed that the Soviets and Eastern Europeans use anabolic-androgenic steroids to help post their remarkable performances on the playing field. They do. These countries' sports federations' reputa-

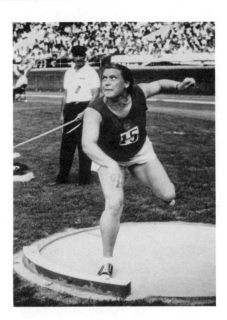

Tamara Press, The Flower of Leningrad, competing at the 1964 Olympic Games. *Note.* © Allsport USA. 1964. Reprinted by permission.

tions for routinely providing such drugs to their athletes were reinforced during the 1976 Olympic Summer Games in Montreal. There, when the head of the East German swimming delegation was asked about the curiously deep voices his women swimmers had, the official wryly responded in a thick accent, ''Ve have come here to svim, not to sing.''

There have been recent examples of how the art of performance enhancing chemistry has grown in Eastern Europe. In the mid-1980s four Canadian weight lifters were caught at the Montreal airport with 22,515 capsules of anabolic-androgenic steroids and 414 vials of testosterone, purchased for next to nothing behind the Iron Curtain.[10] Today, as the Iron Curtain has begun to disappear, I can only assume that the flow of these drugs between East and West will snowball.

We know the Soviets and East Germans used drugs to aid performances on the playing field for years. We must also remember, however, that the appeal of anabolic-androgenic steroids has always been global. Indeed, Western athletes (as exposed in part by the Ben Johnson affair) have always been equally active in the anabolic-androgenic steroid scene.

And they still are.

# 2

# Beyond Humanity

## *Anabolic-Androgenic Steroids*

Anabolic-androgenic steroids are substances some athletes use to gain a competitive edge by increasing their strength and power.

I should first clarify why I refer to these drugs as "anabolic-androgenic steroids" rather than "anabolic steroids" or just "steroids." The adjective *anabolic* refers to constructive metabolism, here specifically to the muscle-building ability of these synthetic hormones. "Andro-," derived from the Greek word root meaning "man" or "male," combines with "-genic," a suffix meaning "producing" or "forming," to create the word *androgenic*, or "male-producing." *Androgenic* thus refers to masculinizing or male hormonal effects.

All anabolic-androgenic steroids (AAS) are derivatives of the natural male hormone testosterone. The main female hormone, on the other hand, is estrogen. Both males and females have varying ratios of these two hormones in their systems, ratios that dictate whether we become male or female. People with a testosterone-dominated hormone balance are male. Those with an estrogen-dominated hormone balance are female.

When I talk about androgenic effects of anabolic-androgenic steroids, I am talking about the masculinizing side effects that may cause health problems among the athletes taking them. For example, the androgenic effects can cause symptoms such as premature baldness, aggressive behavior, and prostate enlargement in males. Remember, prostate gland enlargement was one of the clues Dr. Ziegler used to discover testosterone use by Soviet athletes in the 1950s. Androgenic hormonal effects make these drugs a serious health threat for a variety of other reasons I will discuss later.

First, though, I want to make clear that there is absolutely no anabolic-androgenic steroid that affects an athlete anabolically without also affecting

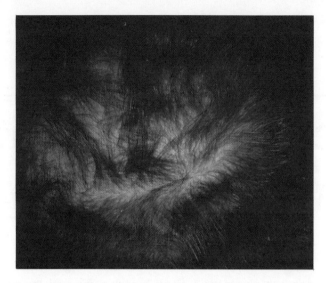

An 18-year-old anabolic-androgenic steroid user showing signs of premature baldness.
*Note.* Photograph courtesy of Dr. Michael J. Scott. Reprinted by permission.

him or her androgenically. Dr. Ziegler failed in his attempt to completely rid these substances of androgenic side effects when he introduced Dianabol, as have all others who have attempted to create a purely anabolic drug. There isn't an anabolic-androgenic steroid an athlete can take to increase muscle mass, endurance, or speed without risking dangerous hormonal side effects.

The point is that the athlete who takes anabolic-androgenic steroids gets the whole package. One effect can't be realized (increased muscle mass, etc.) without the other (male hormonal body changes, etc.). In a sense, given the nature of anabolic-androgenic steroids, athletes can't have their cake and eat it, too. It is important for athletes to know this and equally important for everyone to understand that when someone discusses steroids in sport, they are referring to anabolic-androgenic steroids.

There is another reason to properly identify these drugs. All hormones are, in biochemical terms, steroids. Cortisone, for example, is a steroid. Cortisone and its derivatives are commonly used in sport to reduce inflammation caused by injury. It is also used after surgery. But cortisone is *catabolic*, that is, it may cause muscle destruction and wasting when used over a long period of time. Cortisone has no muscle strengthening effects at all. Athletes may think that when a doctor puts them on a course of cortisone they have been given an anabolic steroid, but this is not the case at all. Some who have tested positive for anabolic-androgenic steroids like to think, or to have others believe, that cortisone is actually what they have tested positive for. But that excuse only works on the ignorant because under medical scrutiny, catabolic steroids and anabolic-androgenic steroids are like apples and oranges.

In addition, it's important to know mixing or combining catabolic and anabolic-androgenic steroids can do some nasty things to the body. In one particular case, I suspect that an American weight lifter had used high doses of anabolic-androgenic steroids and corticosteroids to help prepare for the 1984 Olympic Games. Those drugs had so scrambled the kinetic balance of his muscles that when his thigh muscle straightened while he was trying to lift his maximum in Los Angeles, the huge patellar tendon connected to the lower leg ruptured. The sound of the rupture echoed throughout the auditorium. The tendon, normally a solid, smooth substance, became a stretched-out mass of broken fibers resembling two wet mops end on end.

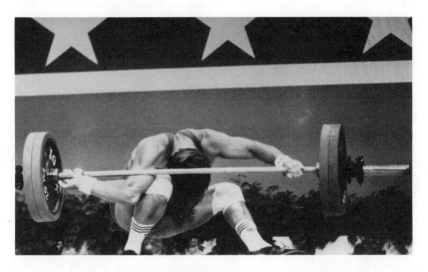

This athlete suffered a dislocated elbow and ruptured patellar tendon—possibly the result of mixing anabolic-androgenic and catabolic steroids.
*Note.* Photograph reprinted by permission of UPI/Bettmann Newsphotos and the Bettmann Archives.

The use and abuse of anabolic-androgenic steroids is one of the most controversial topics in sport today. Athletes often refer to these drugs as "the breakfast of champions," which shows just how prevalent and innocent athletes feel AAS use is. Only after Ben Johnson of Canada was stripped of his gold medal and world record after winning the men's 100-meter dash in the Seoul Olympics did this issue erupt into the headlines of sports pages around the world.

Nonetheless, these drugs have been used by athletes to gain a competitive edge for the better part of 3 decades. Dr. Allan Ryan, Dr. Daniel Hanley, and Dr. William Taylor, all former medical advisors to the USOC, had each spent much time and effort in an attempt to alert the medical profession and the sports community to the abuse of anabolic-androgenic steroids among athletes long before Seoul. But until very recently, no one had really listened. The USOC and the IOC didn't officially ban anabolic-androgenic steroids from competition until before the 1976 Olympic

---

## BANNED ANABOLIC-ANDROGENIC STEROIDS

| Generic name | Example |
| --- | --- |
| Bolasterone | |
| Boldenone | Vebonol, Equipoise |
| Clostebol | Sternabol |
| Dehydrochlormethyl-testosterone | Turnibol |
| Fluoxymesterone, Ultrandren | Android-F, Halotestin, Ora-testryl, |
| Mesterolone | Androviron, Proviron |
| Metandienone | Danabol, Dianabol |
| Metenolone | Primobolan, Primobolan-Depot |
| Methandrostenolone | Dianabol |
| Methyltestosterone | Android, Estratest, Metandren, Oreton, Testred |
| Nandrolone, Nandrobolic | Durabolin, Deca-Durabolin, Kabolin |
| Norethandrolone | Nilevar |
| Oxandrolone | Anavar |
| Oxymesterone | Oranabol, Theranabol |
| Oxymetholone | Anadrol, Nilevar, Anapolon, Adroyd |
| Stanozolol | Winstrol, Stromba |
| Testosterone | Malogen, Malogex, Delatestryl, Oreton |

### . . . and related compounds, e.g.:

| | |
| --- | --- |
| Danazol | Danocrine |
| Growth hormone | |
| Human chorionic gonadotrophin | |
| Zeranol | |

From: U.S. Olympic Committee drug education handbook *Drug Free*, 1989-1992.

Summer Games in Montreal, years after AAS had initially been introduced to athletes.

Anabolic-androgenic steroids are still tremendously popular among a high number of athletes for one simple reason: They work. Any doubters of anabolic-androgenic steroid effects simply needed to watch Ben Johnson blow away the field in the 100-meter dash in Seoul to become believers.

Anabolic-androgenic steroids increase lean muscle mass and strength when used in conjunction with training. It is important to note here that AAS work only in conjunction with an intensive weight training program. AAS can't do anything training and nutrition cannot do, but they can change the body faster than normal. People can't sit on their butts and pop AAS pills and get big! Also, as with any drug, there are positive and negative side effects that may occur. I discuss some of the serious short-term and long-term side effects of anabolic-androgenic steroids later.

Thus, not only are AAS wrong because they can be used to gain an unfair advantage, but they also present the athlete with a terrible health risk—a situation I believe is a doubly unfair predicament. I have known elite, postcollege athletes who have had to decide between taking AAS to have half a chance to effectively compete internationally, and giving up sport altogether rather than risk their health by taking the drugs. That's one of the most salient arguments I know of against lifting the ban on AAS, assuming that every competitor could be given an equal chance and a fair choice.

Unfortunately, the general public thinks anabolic-androgenic steroids are used mainly by football players, weight lifters, and power event participants in track and field. In actuality, however, AAS use is almost universal in sport today. I have seen anabolic-androgenic steroids used by athletes in all running events, swimming, wrestling, cycling, and most team sports. In fact, the only Olympic sports where I have not witnessed AAS use have been table tennis, women's field hockey, men's and women's figure skating, equestrian events, and women's gymnastics. When I'm asked which sports' athletes take steroids, I usually answer, "You show me a sport where increased power, endurance, or speed can possibly benefit the athlete, and I'll show you a sport where AAS use exists."

There are about 25 different derivatives of testosterone that make up the list of available AAS. Basically, anabolic-androgenic steroids come in three forms: (a) the C-17 alkyl derivatives of testosterone; (b) esters (or derivatives) of 19-nortestosterone; and (c) esters of testosterone. It is important to understand the differentiation among these three types.

The C-17 alkyl derivatives of testosterone are anabolic-androgenic steroids that are water soluble and can be taken by mouth. In other words, these anabolic-androgenic steroids are orally active: They're pills. Some examples of C-17 alkyl derivatives include

- methandrostenolone, a.k.a. Dianabol or D-bol;
- oxandrolone, a.k.a. Anavar;
- oxymetholone, a.k.a. Anadrol; and
- stanozolol, a.k.a. Winstrol.

What is important to understand about these forms of AAS is that because they are water soluble and orally active, their clearance times (the time an athlete needs to pass traces of these drugs from the body) are usually quite short, although clearance times do vary depending on the body weight of the user, the dose administered, and the frequency of use. The medical literature on anabolic-androgenic steroids states that most oral forms of these drugs can clear the body in 3 to 4 weeks. Through discussions with many athletes who have used AAS, however, I have learned that the educated user can sometimes clear water-soluble AAS much faster. Recognizing how adept at beating the tests some athletes have become in recent years, I tend to believe it.

The second group of anabolic-androgenic steroids, the esters of 19-nortestosterone, are oil-based, fat soluble, and active when injected into the body. Saying these drugs are fat soluble means that they are absorbed into the body's fat deposits, where long-term energy is stored. When the user mobilizes the body's fat stores by expending energy through exercise, AAS in the system are slowly released and made active. The advantage of this process is a much smoother and effective action of the drug when used in conjunction with intense weight training.

The most popular oil-based anabolic-androgenic steroid is nandrolone, a.k.a. Deca-Durabolin or just Deca. There seems to be little question among users that nandrolone is probably the most effective anabolic-androgenic steroid. The problem with nandrolone, however, is that because it is stored in the fat and released over a longer period, it can sometimes take 6 to 8 months to clear the athlete's system. Nandrolone is the most commonly detected anabolic-androgenic steroid in after-competition drug tests because of this long window of detectability. For this reason, nandrolone becomes a high-risk drug to the athlete who will, at some point, be subjected to drug testing.

I have dealt with problem cases where an athlete has tested positive for nandrolone for as long as 12 months after using this drug. In another case, though I found it hard to believe, an athlete told me after testing positive for nandrolone that he had not taken the drug for 18 months prior to the test. I did have some reason to believe him, although it is virtually impossible to know whether athletes are telling the truth or not about their most recent use.

This potential danger of detection is the reason why *The Underground Steroid Users Handbook*, the anabolic-androgenic steroid users' bible, cautions athletes not to use nandrolone anymore.

---

*Author's Note:   The Underground Steroid Users Handbook* is not a legitimate book. It is a brochure people like me probably aren't supposed to know about. Some drug "gurus" hand these out to their customers. Often, it accompanies black market orders. I know exactly what's in it. And I know athletes refer to it religiously.

---

There is another aspect to this situation, however. The oil-based esters of nandrolone, or 19-nortestosterone, because of their slow release process, probably have the fewest dangerous, androgenic side effects of the three forms of anabolic-androgenic steroids. Because these drugs do not have to be cleared first through the liver, they do not create the risks of liver disease which the oral anabolic-androgenic steroids create.

A sad paradox is that after drug testers and sport federations worldwide have worked so hard to eliminate the AAS problem because of the potential health risks to athletes, we have in a sense steered the athletes toward more dangerous drugs. The types of drug testing programs used by doping control authorities today have unintentionally created a greater health danger in that athletes are now using the shorter acting, more toxic forms of these drugs to avoid detection. Athletes have stopped using nandrolone, which in relative terms is a safe AAS, and are now using the more dangerous orally active forms of AAS, the C-17 alkyl derivatives. In addition, many have gone to using the third, and most dangerous, type of anabolic-androgenic steroids: the esters of testosterone.

The esters (or derivatives) of testosterone are active both orally and by injection. Because testosterone is the natural male hormone, however, when this substance appears in an after-competition urine sample, a drug tester cannot distinguish if the testosterone was supplied naturally by the athlete's body or from an outside, synthetic form of the drug. Commonly used forms of testosterone include testosterone propionate, a.k.a. Testex, and testosterone cypionate.

Drug testing officials have had to formulate a different process to detect synthetic testosterone. In this testing process, a drug laboratory distinguishes a ratio between the testosterone and its free analog, epitestosterone, found in an athlete's urine. Normally, this ratio is 1:1. When foreign testosterone is administered into the body, this ratio rises. The IOC Medical Commission has established a 6:1 testosterone:epitestosterone ratio as abnormal. Anything at or above that cutoff level constitutes a doping violation for testosterone use.

---

*Author's Note:*   In my opinion, this cutoff is high. It allows a "normal" athlete with a 1:1 ratio to boost his or her testosterone to 5.9 times the natural level without fear of breaking the standards. This must change. This area needs research and a realistic cutoff ratio. As it stands, athletes are using testosterone and very little is being done to effectively control the problem.

---

Straight testosterone has the most negative, androgenic side effects of any anabolic substance, and health risks increase with sustained use. Yet the aqueous (water-soluble) forms of testosterone clear the system quite rapidly. Thus, athletes in search of anabolic enhancement along with prevention of detection by urine testing use aqueous testosterone. They are willing to subject themselves to the health risks inherent in testosterone use because this drug is the most effective of its type in avoiding detection.

Just what are the mechanisms of action for AAS? How and why do they work? These are difficult questions to answer because very few detailed, scientific human studies on anabolic-androgenic steroids are available in the medical literature. Anabolic-androgenic steroids seem to reverse the negative or catabolic effects exercise has on muscles (remember, catabolic is the opposite of anabolic: Catabolism breaks down muscle tissue). During exercise the adrenal glands naturally secrete hormones that induce muscle breakdown. Experts believe that anabolic-androgenic steroids actively dampen or minimize this effect and thus build muscle in the absence of muscle deterioration.

There needs to be more understanding of anabolic-androgenic steroids before we can claim these drugs directly stimulate the synthesis of protein, which forms the building blocks for muscle development. Yet some scientists have argued that anabolic-androgenic steroids are indeed capable of enhancing the direct development of muscle fibers by affecting the body's conservation of nitrogen. A positive nitrogen balance facilitates protein buildup and thus an increased rate of muscle production.

Other scientists feel that anabolic-androgenic steroids help the gastrointestinal (digestive) tract better absorb ingested proteins.

Adolph Hitler used testosterone on his troops during World War II to make them more hostile and fearless killers. More is being learned about such psychological, especially the aggression-inducing, effects of anabolic-androgenic steroids. Through elicitation of "macho" behavior, testosterone makes an athlete train harder, and because of the positive nitrogen balance, the athlete recovers from exercise quicker; the athlete gains muscle mass accordingly. Increased frequency and intensity of training is the key to muscle strength and development.

Why don't we know more about anabolic-androgenic steroids, however? In an era of heart transplants, why can't the medical profession figure these drugs out? This lack of simple, certain answers is one of the reasons physicians have lost a substantial amount of credibility with athletes.

Because physicians couldn't offer scientific facts about how anabolic-androgenic steroids worked when these drugs were initially introduced, some doctors suggested that their effects were probably only psychological. Athletes who could gain 25 to 30 pounds of lean muscle mass and lift 25 to 30 percent more weight within just 10 to 12 weeks of using anabolic-androgenic steroids, of course, knew there was more to these drugs than mere psychological, placebo effects. Hence, a lot of athletes who used AAS thought doctors didn't know what they were talking about.

Even today, this communication gap remains a major factor in our inability to convince athletes that AAS are harmful. Physicians can't relate authoritatively to this subject due to the lack of adequate human research. The reasons scientific research still can't be done effectively are: (a) human experimentation committees, which judge whether to approve any human research study, allow investigation with only therapeutic doses, which are much smaller than those used by athletes to build muscle; and (b) the drugs work so well it is hard to mask the lack of effects when the control substance or placebo is given.

The problem in the first case is that athletes use AAS in far higher doses than those considered safe by legitimate therapeutic standards. Athletes often use multiple forms of anabolic-androgenic steroids, "stacking" one form of the drug on another in regimens called cycles. These cycles are individually tailored by experienced steroid gurus.

A sample cycle might be 12 weeks in length, with the athlete using aqueous testosterone, 1/4 to 1 cc per day; and Winstrol (stanozolol) oral tablets daily, with a 5-mg incremental increase each week for 5 weeks before a gradual tapered reduction. The whole cycle may be initially stimulated with several hundred milligrams of nandrolone. In the final 3 or 4 weeks of the cycle, when Winstrol use might taper, aqueous testosterone doses might be increased. Human chorionic gonadotrophin (HCG), which stimulates the body's natural production of testosterone, would then be given to restart the body's normal production of testosterone, which was shut down during the cycle.

There are numerous variations of this cycle, some substituting Anavar for Winstrol, others adding an anti-estrogen such as tamoxifen citrate (Nolvadex) to combat aromatization, a process by which the body metabolizes and gets rid of the tremendous doses. Aromatization converts testosterone to estrogen (a female hormone). This excess estrogen circulating in the bloodstream leads to some fascinating side effects, which will be discussed later.

One can see from the foregoing that any self-respecting body of scientists or doctors would never agree to this type of drug dosing on humans for research purposes, even though there *are* athletes willing to participate in such testing. Despite the fact that research is difficult to come by, I believe we *must* continue our search for answers on this subject. Unfortunately, sport officials and many scientists are not committed to discovering alternative ways to research AAS. Thus, athletes are taking these drugs as the sports and scientific communities sit idly by. I think a great deal of research could be obtained through working with the user-athletes themselves, but, obviously this is a difficult hurdle to cross. How can we expect to obtain information from user-athletes on this subject when most of the drug control resources in this country are funneled into testing programs with witch-hunt mentalities?

Another reason solid research is difficult to come by is the very effectiveness of these drugs and their profound physical and psychological effects. To study a drug, most researchers choose to give one group of their test volunteers the real drug and another group a placebo. In some cases, researchers may choose to give a third group a different drug altogether. This has to be done in such a way that the subjects have no idea which drug they are being given. After observing the effects of the various substances on the different groups, the drugs are switched for comparative purposes. This is called a double-blind crossover study, and to date it is the only scientifically acceptable method for proving a drug action.

Because anabolic-androgenic steroids are so effective, though, it is hard to find a placebo or another substance that subjects would take and not know they weren't getting the real thing. Therefore, it is impossible to gauge how many of these drugs' effects are physiological and how many are psychological.

Dr. Irving Dardik, former chairman of the USOC Sports Medicine Council, used to explain how we might be able to get around this dilemma. He suggested we train a laboratory rat or cat to throw a javelin or shot put. Then, with these subjects we could once and for all prove not only how the drugs work but if they are indeed able to improve strength and performance. Admittedly, this is a facetious proposition, but it is one of the few possibilities at hand.

So much for how these drugs work for athletes. In legitimate medical practice there are only a few specific, uncommon therapeutic uses for anabolic-androgenic steroids. These include stimulation of the bone marrow in certain patients with a very rare anemia, stimulation of sexual development in boys with low testicular production of testosterone, a possible palliative treatment for terminal breast cancer patients, and treatment of a rare condition known as hereditary angioedema (which is caused by an inherited enzyme deficiency).

The incidence of these uncommon cases makes medical use of AAS rare. In fact, many pharmaceutical companies have stopped making these drugs because of their limited value in legitimate practice. An interesting rumor is that CIBA, the manufacturer of methandrostenolone (Dianabol), recently researched the purposes their drug was used for. They found that most users of the drug were athletes and that very little methandrostenolone was used for medical purposes. Consequently, they halted its manufacture.

There is, of course, another reason drug firms have limited or stopped production of anabolic-androgenic steroids. These drugs were initially produced for their theorized ability to synthesize protein. These drugs did offer some limited benefits to cancer patients and burn victims, who because of skin loss become protein deficient. However, the side effects experienced by the patients using these substances created more problems than they solved. Side effects such as increased blood pressure, heart disease, and liver cancer, to name a few, far outweighed the benefits.

This is an important point. Athletes today are skeptical of the medical profession's cautions about bad side effects from anabolic-androgenic steroid use. Yet, despite the little amount of research and information available to physicians, we are well aware from the documented cases that the side effects are real. Additionally, many of us who have followed athletes using AAS have seen the harmful side effects. Athletes need to know this. Physicians and health authorities do know what they're talking about when they discuss the potential dangers of anabolic-androgenic steroids.

The harmful effects of anabolic-androgenic steroids have been described in various ways by many. In working directly with athletes, I have seen a wide spectrum of side effects resulting from anabolic-androgenic steroids.

I have not witnessed liver cancer, kidney tumors, heart attacks, or death among anabolic-androgenic steroid users. I hope I never do, for AAS have indeed been attributed to well-documented cases of such problems, cases I will describe shortly. In addition, I want it understood that I'm not an alarmist. People aren't continually dropping over dead from the use of AAS. In fact, alcohol claims far more lives in one year alone than AAS will in a decade. But death *is* a possible result of anabolic-androgenic steroid use.

Health effects are only one part of the issue at hand. We should not forget that a second complication of AAS use among athletes is that fair competition is not possible. Even if these drugs did not produce harmful side effects, we would still have to ban them if we wanted fair and equal competition.

Some of the aforementioned physical effects go away once the user stops taking anabolic-androgenic steroids. Others—such as male baldness, impotence; female hair growth, deepening of the voice, enlargement of the clitoris; the scarring of cystic acne, certain psychological changes, and stunted growth—are irreversible and permanent.

## SIDE EFFECTS FROM ANABOLIC-ANDROGENIC STEROID USE

- Acne: serious cystic types that leave permanent scars on the face, body, and trunk
- Nervous tension, aggressiveness, and psychotic states; paranoia; and antisocial behavior
- Increased sex drive after initial use, but decreased sex drive after repeated use (often leading to psychologically caused impotence)
- Breast development in males, also known as gynecomastia (a permanent effect)
- Gastrointestinal and leg muscle cramping
- Headaches, dizziness, and high blood pressure
- Burning and pain while urinating
- Bizarre testicular or scrotal pain
- Premature male baldness (particularly alarming among 17-year-olds)
- Excessive body and facial hair growth among women
- Atrophy of testicles and decreased sperm production
- Prostate enlargement, causing urination to be difficult
- Enlargement of the clitoris, the female organ analogous to the male penis (usually irreversible and may require surgical removal)
- Disruption of the menstrual cycle
- Deepening of the voice (permanent in women)
- Stunted growth among adolescents, basically due to premature stoppage of the expected growth of long bones

I think it is both interesting and instructive to explain some of these bizarre reactions in detail. Take, for example, gynecomastia, feminine breast development among men using anabolic-androgenic steroids. Why do these muscular, macho men taking AAS develop female breasts, or bitch tits, as they are commonly referred to in the muscle building gyms? (By the way, once these breasts form, they are in most cases permanent. Of course, men find growing female breasts cosmetically unacceptable and eventually must undergo surgery to have them removed.) Such development is rather complicated biologically and physiologically, but maybe I can simplify.

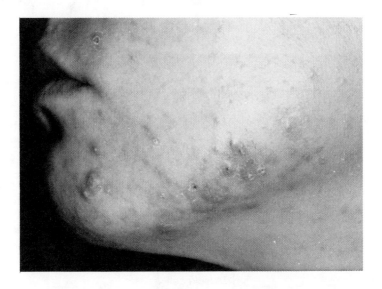

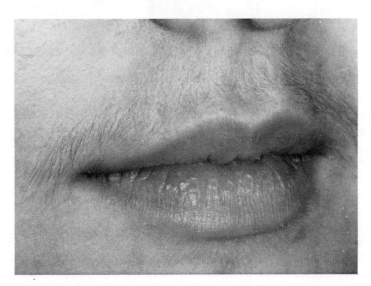

Examples of side effects of anabolic-androgenic steroid use: a) cystic acne;
b) female facial hair growth.
*Note.* Photographs courtesy of Dr. Michael J. Scott. Reprinted by permission.

Fooling around with the body's hormone system is a dangerous
business. Our hormonal balance is based on a cyclic feedback mechanism
(see Figure 1). The hypothalamus, in the brain, is the regulator. It sends
signals to the master gland, the pituitary, at the base of the brain. The

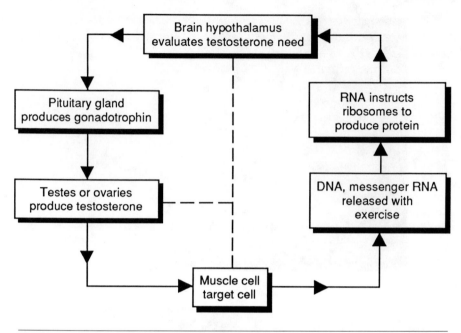

**Figure 1.** The feedback mechanism on which the human hormonal balance is based.

pituitary gland's hormones stimulate target organs such as the thyroid, testicles, ovaries, and adrenal glands. These produce their own hormones, which circulate in the bloodstream to be used by various target cells when and where needed.

Any interruption of this cycle by inserting testosterone not produced by the body causes the hypothalamus to recognize no further need to produce testosterone. Hence, it shuts down the body's testosterone manufacturing process. This completely disrupts normal hormonal ratios and causes a communications break with DNA and messenger RNA functions, which in turn can sometimes cause bizarre side effects such as atrophy of the testes in a male and, in this case, the development of breasts.

Another example is what may happen in an adolescent using anabolic-androgenic steroids. Receptors in bones responsible for bone growth react to the surplus testosterone circulating in the bloodstream. These receptors become saturated and further growth ceases. The growth centers then fuse permanently, and the youngster may never achieve the growth in stature planned by the body's genes. The adolescent may grow wider but not taller, a condition often seen among weight lifters who started anabolic-androgenic steroid use before reaching maturity.

The detrimental effects anabolic-androgenic steroids have on the liver are also quite complicated; they mainly involve the orally active AAS, such as the derivatives Dianabol, Anavar, Anadrol, and stanozolol. The oral AAS must be metabolized by the liver. Athletes use toxically high doses that cause destruction of liver cells in a way similar to what happens in hepatitis. Such liver toxicity is characterized by symptoms such as nausea, vomiting, and jaundice. Continued anabolic-androgenic steroid use can lead to more significant liver cell destruction and a condition called peliosis hepatitis, or degeneration of liver tissue into blood-filled cysts. These cysts can become quite large and may rupture and bleed. A 27-year-old British bodybuilder recently bled to death, despite surgical efforts to save his life, after a blood cyst in his liver ruptured.

Cases of liver cancer among sick patients or burn victims who received anabolic-androgenic steroid therapy have been well documented. In one study of 36 cases of liver tumors, C-17 alkyl anabolic-androgenic steroids (orally active) had been used over a course of months to years in each case. Seven of the tumors were innocent, or benign, but 29 were cancerous, or malignant. The benign tumors were attributed to 6 to 24 months of C-17 alkyl anabolic-androgenic steroid use. The malignant cases were each attributed to more than 24 months of use. And remember, the doses given to these patients were lower than the doses some athletes are using.

There have been only a few reported cases of liver cancer among athletes who used anabolic-androgenic steroids. For example, in March 1984 bodybuilder Daniel Baroudi died of liver cancer at the age of 26. His illness was believed to have been brought on by his 4-year involvement with C-17 alkyl derivative anabolic-androgenic steroids.

Heart and circulatory diseases are other side effects of anabolic-androgenic steroids that occur after long-term use—sort of a time bomb effect, if you will. Several well-documented studies now show that anabolic-androgenic steroid use may lead to premature arteriosclerosis, or hardening of the arteries. This, in turn, can lead to damage of the heart, the brain, and the kidneys.

Premature arteriosclerosis is believed to be due to the effect anabolic-androgenic steroids have on lowering the body's level of high density lipoproteins (HDLs), the beneficial blood lipid (fat) that protects against cholesterol buildup in the arteries. A lowered level of HDLs provokes premature atherosclerosis or clogging of the arteries with cholesterol, which we commonly see among older individuals but certainly don't expect to see among 17- to 25-year-olds. This aging process leads to high blood pressure and, potentially, heart attacks or strokes. This would seem to be a high price to pay at a young age for a few years of fame and glory on the athletic field.

One athlete who is paying such a price is former Pittsburgh Steeler lineman Steve Courson, who is suffering from cardiomyopathy, which describes a deteriorating heart. He is now on the waiting list for a heart transplant. I have heard that Courson's resting heart rate was, at one time, well over 100 beats per minute. Courson, along with a variety of experts in this field, thinks his religious use of anabolic-androgenic steroids during his professional football career may have contributed greatly to his present condition.

Another case of heart disease, this time fatal, attributed to anabolic-androgenic steroid use was that of high school football player Benji Ramirez. Ramirez, of Ashtabula, Ohio, died of a heart attack on October 31, 1988. On January 10, 1989, County Coroner Dr. Robert Malinkowski issued an official statement saying that this young man's death was in part attributable to his use of anabolic-androgenic steroids.

Steven Vallie, a former high school football standout and bodybuilder from New Haven, Connecticut, died of heart failure in the Phoenix Gym in New Haven on March 19, 1989. Vallie's autopsy revealed that his athlete's heart was enlarged and scarred, probably due to his use of anabolic-androgenic steroids. Vallie was 21.

Former bodybuilder Glenn Mauer suffered a stroke in 1983 at the age of 33. One month later he had to undergo a quadruple bypass operation. Mauer's religious use of anabolic-androgenic steroids caused his deteriorated health.

Larry Pacifico, a nine-time American powerlifting champion, was similarly forced to undergo a quadruple coronary bypass operation at the age of 35. His condition was also brought on by anabolic-androgenic steroid use.

Cindy Olavarri, a member of the United States 1984 Olympic Cycling Team, today suffers severe muscle and joint stiffness, a deepened voice, psychological problems, and particular sensitivity to infections. She has publicly attributed this to her use of anabolic-androgenic steroids during her athletic career.[11]

Despite the severity of these physical health risks, perhaps the greatest dangers associated with anabolic-androgenic steroid use are the psychological effects these drugs have on the user. The psychological changes brought on by AAS include aggressiveness and feelings of indestructibility and power. Although the advantages these feelings bring on the playing field may be considerable, the athlete cannot turn these feelings off once the competition is over. Consequently, AAS often serve to harm the user or others.

Physiology studies on the limbic area of the brain have identified androgen receptors that cause similar effects to appear when stimulated electrically. Some informal reports indicate that the higher the dose of anabolic-androgenic steroids, the more aggressive the user becomes. There doesn't appear to be a limit to the amount an individual might change. This syndrome closely resembles the classic Dr. Jekyll and

Mr. Hyde personality. The more androgenic the drugs are, the greater the personality change. Straight testosterone seems to be the worst offender in this category, with Anadrol, Anavar, and Dianabol following, in that order.

I have seen mood swings, increased libido, sexual perversion, violent, uncontrollable behavior, and even psychotic episodes among athletes who used anabolic-androgenic steroids. Minor and temporary behavior changes, though potentially dangerous, may occur while an athlete is on an anabolic-androgenic drug cycle. These episodes of uncontrolled aggressive behavior, described as "roid rage," are fairly common among anabolic-androgenic steroid users. I have heard from girlfriends and wives of AAS users the fears they have when their boyfriends and spouses are "cycling" on these drugs. Relationships are often strained because of insatiable and often aggressive appetites for sex brought on by AAS.

Roid rage is common among women as well as men. Tina Plakinger, a 32-year-old former national bodybuilding champion, has related how she grabbed her husband and forcefully jacked him up against a wall one night. The reason? He was late for dinner.

Believe it or not, such extreme reactions are fairly common among anabolic-androgenic steroid users. Roid rage, or, as it is also called, anabolic madness, is not new. This effect of anabolic-androgenic steroids has been observed for some time.

Harrison Pope, Jr., MD, and David Katz, MD, of Harvard University recently reported a study of 41 anabolic-androgenic steroid users. They found 12 percent of their subjects were overtly psychotic, 10 percent were subthreshold psychotic, 30 percent suffered major mood swings, and 12 percent experienced manic episodes. Symptoms noted in their review included hallucinations, paranoia, explosive behavior, grandiose beliefs, "Superhuman complex," mania, and irritability.

I have personally seen numerous cases of psychotic behavior among athletes who used anabolic-androgenic steroids. These athletes seem to lose all regard for safety. They hallucinate, walk in front of moving cars, and inflict severe pain on themselves and others—all because anabolic-androgenic steroids have so seriously warped their thoughts and emotions.

I flinched when the infamous Oklahoma football player Brian Bosworth was found positive for anabolic-androgenic steroids by NCAA drug testing before the Orange Bowl in December 1986. His coach, now former Oklahoma coach, Barry Switzer, naively stated that he was, at least, thankful that The Boz wasn't positive for cocaine. The implication was that cocaine, unlike anabolic-androgenic steroids, is a bad, mind-influencing drug. But, truth be known, anabolic-androgenic steroids can be equally mind influencing. Aggressive and even psychotic behavior, which everyone knows is what made The Boz famous to begin with, is, I suppose, safer on a football field than when directed at a girlfriend or a spouse. The problem is that the athlete can't switch these feelings off on the way home from the stadium. Thus, one really has to worry about the potential harm to society by persons cycling on anabolic-androgenic steroids.

Several court cases have considered the effects of anabolic-androgenic steroids on the defendants' behavior. David Williams, an alleged burglar and arsonist, was arrested and tried in 1986 in the first case, to my knowledge, that addressed whether anabolic-androgenic steroids can induce criminal behavior and, if so, whether being under the influence of AAS is a legitimate legal defense. The judge opined that the defendant "was suffering from an organic personality syndrome caused by toxic levels of anabolic steroids taken to enhance his ability to win body building contests."[12] In other words, Williams received a diminished response verdict for using anabolic-androgenic steroids.

While acting as a drug control officer for the U.S. Olympic Committee, Dr. Thomas B. Dickson testified in a case where a male weight lifter and bodybuilder in his early 20s, while taking the anabolic-androgenic steroids Dianabol, Winstrol V, Deca-Durabolin, and testosterone, violently beat to death a fellow bodybuilder who made a provocative homosexual pass at him while they were having a drink at a local pub.

A veteran highway patrolman in Oregon, while using anabolic-androgenic steroids to maintain his bulk, shot and paralyzed a female store clerk for making an innocent but mildly offensive remark after he had asked to use her telephone.

In Boca Raton, Florida, an AAS user robbed and murdered a man whose body was found hanging from two stakes.

A Louisiana high school football player who used AAS killed a couple in their home during a botched burglary attempt.

Other cases have described how anabolic-androgenic steroids may actually lead an athlete to self-destruction. Michael Keys, a young Mt. Clemens, Michigan, resident, committed suicide while experiencing the psychological effects of the drugs he was taking, as did a young Kansas City, Missouri, weight lifter. Many have heard the story reported in *Sports Illustrated* of former University of South Carolina noseguard Tommy Chaikin, who nearly blew his brains out because of AAS.

These types of stories are being reported over and over again. My fear is that we have here a drug with as much potential for harm to the individual, and possibly society, as any drug that exists. Not many people or even professionals realize this.

Another danger associated with anabolic-androgenic steroids is their addictive capability. Anabolic-androgenic steroids have been connected with both physiological and psychological addiction. The mechanisms of physiological addiction are quite easy to understand. Using anabolic-androgenic steroids causes the body to shut off its normal hypothalamic-pituitary-testicular feedback mechanisms. When the athlete stops using anabolic-androgenic steroids, a period of withdrawal sets in because the body no longer produces its own testosterone. Until the body cranks up its production of testosterone, muscle and abdominal cramps, lethargy, constipation, headaches, and reactive depression may occur. If this is not countered with psychological counseling and possibly antidepressant medication, the athlete either starts another cycle of the drug or turns to amphetamines or other stimulants to make him feel better—sources of other potential addictions. Someone who gets in the habit of taking uppers to get high and downers to relax and come down may get hooked into other forms of drug addiction.

To understand AAS addiction, one must understand how these very effective muscle building drugs change the person's basic physical and psychological characteristics. Remember the old advertisements on the back of comic books that touted the Charles Atlas muscle program? In these ads, the 90-pound weakling gets sand kicked in his face by the muscle man on the beach. After taking the Charles Atlas dynamic muscle building course for just a few months, however, the weakling suddenly blossoms into a hulking, macho muscle man, never again to be ridiculed on the beach.

Now, I'm not sure how well the old Charles Atlas course actually worked, but I know anabolic-androgenic steroids can get the same job done in a few short months. For example, a 130-pound youngster who starts using anabolic-androgenic steroids can, in a matter of weeks, realize an additional 30 or 40 pounds or more of bulging, cut (no-fat) muscle. Not only will he look better in his muscle shirt, but he'll feel more confident. He'll have an increased sex drive, and he won't feel shy around the girls or in the gym where he works out.

Unfortunately, in order to maintain his newfound macho personality and Charles Atlas body, he must continue taking anabolic-androgenic steroids. The instant he stops, the majority of the gains he's made will begin to melt away. He can't face that possibility: He can't be small again and lose the respect and stature he's grown to enjoy. Hence, he feels compelled to continue using anabolic-androgenic steroids.

This type of addiction often begins at an early age, when most youngsters are already experiencing an identity crisis. For many, once they've started on anabolic-androgenic steroids, there's no going back. This psychological dependency is probably the worst form of addiction. It's one thing in sport, where the aggression can be played out on the field, but it's another thing when the addiction sets in among youngsters who don't care as much about performance enhancement as about being big and strong, an identity the average young man could find hard to give up.

This is particularly disturbing when one considers the 1989 study published by Buckley, Yesalis, Friedl, Anderson, Streit, and Wright in the

*Journal of the American Medical Association.* These researchers discovered that 6.6 percent of the high school seniors they sampled used anabolic-androgenic steroids. Over two thirds of these students had tried them before the age of 16. Interestingly, 47.7 percent of these students used AAS to enhance athletic performance, whereas 26.7 percent used them solely to improve appearance. In fact, 35.7 percent of the users were not involved in organized school sports whatsoever.[13] These figures lent credence to a previous report, by Charles Stebbins of the National Federation of State High School Associations, showing that 18 percent of male high school students in South Plantation, Florida, had used anabolic-androgenic steroids. This is a dangerous trend among young people and one reason I think the drugs need to be better controlled by testing at the high school level.

Anabolic-androgenic steroids are also tremendously popular among female athletes. AAS affect women more profoundly than men. When intense weight training and exercises are maintained, a smaller amount of the drug will create gains for females greater than those experienced by males.

This, to me, is a sad commentary on efforts to equalize the opportunities for women in sport, à la Title IX. Today we no longer have women competing against women, but chemically induced males, or androgynous hermaphrodites, competing against normal women—obviously unequal competition.

In recent years, experts have begun to see even more negative side effects sprouting up among anabolic-androgenic steroid users. There is increasing evidence that continued anabolic-androgenic steroid use (a) increases the risk of muscle ruptures and tears (this happens because of the tremendous hypertrophy and strength in the muscle); (b) increases the possibility of rupturing muscle tendons at the point of insertion into bone; and, because of an increase in body testosterone, (c) blocks the release of calcium across the bone cell membrane, which can lead to a decrease in bone density and increasing brittleness. This is believed to be accountable for the increase in the number of stress fractures seen in many sports today.

It has recently been shown that anabolic-androgenic steroid use can lead to a decrease in the body's immune mechanisms. Leonard H. Calabrese, DO, reported in the February 1988 issue of *Clinical Immunology* that 23 bodybuilders on anabolic-androgenic steroids showed a marked decrease in immunoglobulins, compared to 25 sedentary persons.

This becomes really frightening when you consider that the highest risk group for contracting AIDS (acquired immune deficiency syndrome) is intravenous drug users, not homosexuals. Indeed, several cases of AIDS among AAS-using bodybuilders have already been reported.[14]

Yet the appetite for AAS in this country continues to grow. After the Ben Johnson affair erupted in 1988, I took part in a joint project with *USA Today* while working with the USOC. We established a drug hotline to field calls from across the country on this issue of drugs in sport. Amazingly, most of the calls we received weren't from people concerned about the side effects of AAS or interested in the role these drugs play in various sport competitions, but from people who wanted to know where they could get some of what Ben Johnson took.

Medical professionals and law enforcement officials alike need to address this problem and assume the responsibility for controlling it. As long as people believe that anabolic-androgenic steroids can make them grow bigger and stronger, and as long as they fail to fully understand the dangerous side effects of these drugs, the need for medical control will continue.

Many amateur sport federations and professional sport associations have launched highly publicized, aggressive testing programs to halt anabolic-androgenic steroid use among athletes. But are they really *controlling* the problem?

Don't bet on it.

# 3
# Ups and Downs

## Speed, Narcotics, Beta-Blockers, and Diuretics

Steroids might be the hot topic in sports pages these days, but believe me, there are a whole slew of other drugs athletes can and do use to gain the competitive advantage. The use of stimulants, narcotics, beta-blockers, and diuretics is just as commonplace and just as threatening to the concept of fair play as the use of anabolic-androgenic steroids. Athletes, coaches, and, most of all, sport officials have to realize this. Though drug testing has done a pretty good job of controlling these drugs, this problem certainly hasn't gone away.

### STIMULANTS

Amphetamine and its derivatives ephedrine, phenylpropanolamine, and others—along with caffeine and cocaine—are among the most common central nervous system stimulants used by athletes who hope to gain some illegal competitive edge. These drugs give an athlete a feeling of reduced fatigue and increased aggressiveness and hostility, which can be used to enhance the feeling of competitiveness.

Stimulants are used in a vast variety of sports by all types of athletes who hope to gain an extra boost for competition. I have seen speed used not only by football players, track-and-field athletes, boxers, and basketball players, but even by wrestlers, jockeys, and other athletes who need to meet weight requirements and rely on the anorexic (appetite-suppressant) effects of stimulants to help them lose weight before competing.

## BANNED STIMULANTS

| Generic name | Example |
|---|---|
| Amfepramone | Apisate, Tenuate, Tepanil |
| Amfetaminil | AN 1 (Germany) |
| Amiphenazole | Dapti, Daptazole, Amphisol |
| Amphetamine | Delcobese, Obetrol, Benzedrine, Dexedrine |
| Bemegride | Megimide |
| Benzphetamine | Didrex |
| Caffeine | |
| Cathine | (Norpseudoephedrine) Adiposetten (Germany) |
| Chlorphentermine | Pre-sate, Lucofen |
| Clobenzorex | Dinintel (France) |
| Clorprenaline | Vortel, Asthone (Japanese) |
| Cocaine | Surfacaine |
| Cropropamide | component of Micoren |
| Crotetamide | component of Micoren |
| Diethylpropion HCl | Tenuate, Tepanil |
| Dimetamfetamine | Amphetamine |
| Ephedrine, pseudoephedrine** | Tedral, Bronkotabs, Rynatuss, Primatene |
| Etafedrine | Mercodal, Decapryn, Nethamine |
| Etamivan | Emivan, Vandid |
| Etilamfetamine | Apetinil (Netherlands) |
| Fencamfamin | Envitrol, Altimina, Phencamine |
| Fenetylline | Captagon (Germany) |
| Fenproporex | Antiobes Retard (Spain), Appeitzugler (Germany) |
| Furfenorex | Frugal (Argentina), Frugalan (Spain) |
| Isoetarine | Bronkosol, Bronkometer, Numotac, Dilabron |
| Isoproterenol | Isuprel, Norisodrine, Medihaler-Iso |
| Meclofenoxate | Lucidryl, Brenal |
| Mefenorex | Doracil (Argentina), Pondinil (Switzerland), Rondimen (Germany) |
| Metaproterenol | Alupen, Metaprel |
| Methamphetamine | Desoxyn, Met-Ampi |
| Methoxyphenamine | Ritalin, Orthoxicol Cough Syrup |
| Methylamphetamine | Desoxyn, Met-Ampi |
| Methylephedrine | Tybraine, Methep (Germany, Great Britain) |

| Generic name | Example |
| --- | --- |
| Methylphenidate HCl | Ritalin |
| Morazone | Rosimon-Neu (Germany) |
| Nikethamide | Coramine |
| Pemoline | Cylert, Deltamine, Stimul |
| Pentetrazole | Leptazol |
| Phendimetrazine | Bontril, Plegine |
| Phenmetrazine | Preludin |
| Phentermine HCl | Adipex, Fastin, Ionamin |
| Phenylpropanolamine** | Simutab, Contac, Dexatri, Alka Seltzer Plus |
| Picrotoxin | Cocculin |
| Pipradrol | Meratran, constituent of Alertonic |
| Prolintane | Villescon, Promotil, Katovit |
| Propylhexedrine** | Benzedrex Inhaler |
| Pyrovalerone | Centroton, Thymergix |
| Strychnine | Movellan (Germany) |

**. . . and related compounds.**

*Caffeine: 12 mcg/ml in the urine = Positive test.
**Common ingredient in decongestant cold and sinus medicines.

From: U.S. Olympic Commitee drug education handbook *Drug Free*, 1989-1992.

## *Amphetamines*

As I have mentioned, amphetamines got their initial use among athletes after they were introduced during World War II. Amphetamines first became popular among truck drivers, college students who needed to study for exams, and entertainers. These drugs were also readily accepted by the sports world. Athletes were lured to amphetamines because they felt these drugs would increase their energy, alertness, and speed. Later, athletes also began using various amphetamine derivatives to increase their staying power in endurance sports.

Though scientific studies do not give us any definite conclusions about how well stimulants can enhance performance, we do know these drugs act to stimulate the central nervous system and increase the heart rate, blood pressure, metabolism, and body temperature. My personal opinion is that the popularity of these stimulants among athletes is a fair reflection of their effectiveness on the playing field, despite the lack of scientific proof. This lack of concrete evidence to verify or nullify the claims of drug effects on performance is a problem characteristic of almost every drug abused in sport.

Scientists just do not have the ability to study drugs and performance enhancement in detail, but athletes do. Through experience, I've learned that when an athlete tells me he's taking a drug because it works, I should believe him.

Sports medicine experts do know that stimulants enhance self-confidence, delay fatigue, and increase aggressiveness. Stimulants may also mask pain. The drug thus poses the danger of causing injury or aggravating an already serious injury. Combined with the psychodynamic effects of creating a false sense of greater ability and a loss of judgment, these factors lead to a warped sense of power that may result in accidents to the user and his opponents. For example, boxers can inject their knuckles with Novocain so that the pain of hitting is reduced, thereby allowing for an uninhibited and powerful blow. I once treated a high school football player who used a combination of amphetamine and codeine (a narcotic painkiller) to cover up the pain of a cracked leg bone for 2 weeks of practice and competition—only to have his leg finally shatter while sprinting and dodging a would-be tackler on his way into the end zone. The fracture involved the crack in the big bone of his lower leg (tibia) and also the second bone (fibula), creating a compound (bone protruding through the skin) and comminuted (multiple-fragment) fracture. The complications almost cost him his leg, and he never competed again.

During the 1960s and 1970s, amphetamine use among football players appeared to reach epidemic proportion. My first professional contact with the use of amphetamines among athletes came in the 1970s while I was working in the World Football League (WFL). I learned from certain players how they used amphetamines, also called speed, to get up for a game. There were often "candy jars" filled with amphetamine tablets in the training room. After suiting up, players would literally choke down a handful of these pills as they headed out the tunnel onto the field.

For some, this quick fix became standard practice in their pregame preparation. Not only did the amphetamine tablets help the players mask the pain they might have been feeling before and after kickoff, but they also helped them get psyched. In a sense, the drug amphetamine helped them put their game faces on.

For instance, I used to see players swallow a dozen amphetamine pills right before game time and then play for 3 hours with absolutely no ability to sense pain or inhibition. Sometimes they would come back into the locker room with their arms dripping with blood or with their cracked fingers dangling limply. Of course, these injuries weren't all that interesting or unique—that's football. What was interesting was that a given player could break his finger in two in the first quarter and not realize anything was wrong until he noticed it sticking out at a funny angle when he was taking off his cleats after the game—that's speed.

It was in the WFL that I also first became acquainted with other drugs used by athletes. As a naive physician, I found myself shooting up players with vitamin $B_{12}$ and cortisone on a daily basis. I also got my first exposure to anabolic-androgenic steroids in those years. It didn't take long for me to get a quick education on what doping was all about. At this time, one might remember, shooting up and pill popping were considered just "questionable" medical practice. It would still take a few years before any significant findings related to doping would begin to appear in the medical literature.

Then came the famous 1981 report *The Sunday Syndrome*, by A.J. Mandell, K.D. Stewart, and P.V. Russo, which first publicly exposed the problem of amphetamine abuse in the NFL. Dr. Mandell's report was based on his experiences while working with the San Diego Chargers.

Most team doctors like myself were, at this time, learning the difference between professional and amateur athletes with regard to the need to play with pain at all costs to the body. On the high school level, a physician almost never let an athlete compete if the athlete was suffering from even the most minor injury or if the athlete was feeling any pain or discomfort. On the professional level, however, the physician's job was to do whatever it took to get the athlete back into the game. The professional football player *had* to stay in there. The game was his livelihood, and there was always a lineup of rookies waiting like vultures for him not to return. Therefore, the pro player would beg, borrow, or steal and let the physician do everything in his power to get him in next week's game. From what my colleagues tell me, this situation still hasn't changed that much.

My real-world education on doping and athletes grew after I left the WFL to work on the periphery of the National Basketball Association (NBA) as an assistant to Robert Cook, MD, the team physician for the Portland Trailblazers. There, once again, I observed the abuse of medication and drugs by athletes. Speed is a very popular drug among basketball players, who endure lengthy, tiresome road trips, sometimes playing three or four games a week. Amphetamines were as popular among basketball players as they were among football players in the 1970s.

### Cocaine

Amphetamine use gradually diminished as a new drug of choice, cocaine, came into vogue in the late 1970s. Cocaine quickly rose through the ranks as the stimulant of choice among professional athletes. This drug is indeed more powerful, and it creates more euphoric feelings than amphetamine does. By the mid-1980s, names such as John Drew, Spencer Haywood, Eddie Johnson, Bernard King, John Lucas, and David Thompson (all NBA stars); Monte Bennett, Cliff Branch, Ross Browner, Carl Eller, Thomas Henderson, Dexter Manley, Eugene "Mercury" Morris, George Rogers, Lawrence Taylor, and Art Whittington (NFL players); Willie Aikens, Joaquin Andujar, Steve Bedrosian, Dale Berra, Vida Blue, Juan Bonilla, Enos Cabell, Dick Davis, Dwight Gooden, Keith Hernandez, Steve Howe, Lamarr Hoyt, J.R. Richard, and Alan Wiggins (Major League Baseball players); Steve Durbano, Mark Heaslip, Don Murdoch, Borje Salming, and Derek Sanderson (National Hockey League players); and others began appearing in national sports headlines in connection with cocaine abuse.[15]

The list of cocaine users has multiplied since that time. In fact, the majority of sports feature stories run in this nation's newspapers in the '80s were in some way related to the topic of drug abuse, and the substance most discussed was cocaine. Thus, today almost everyone realizes how huge the cocaine epidemic has become.

Cocaine appeals to athletes in many ways. As a stimulant, it can help them get hyped for a game. Cocaine, like amphetamine, masks pain, and it can provoke feelings of aggression and competitiveness. Yet, away from the game, cocaine is widely used as a recreational drug. The euphoric feelings and intense rush of excitement caused by cocaine use have given this drug appeal throughout all sectors of society. In fact, William Bennett, former secretary of education and now National Drug Policy Director in the Bush administration, lists cocaine as the most dangerous and formidable foe in the nation's new war on drugs. Former Surgeon General C. Everett Koop listed the cocaine crisis as one of the United States' most dangerous, widespread epidemics.

Some elite-level athletes find an emptiness in their lives once they reach the top simply because they feel they have little left to accomplish. Many of them turn to drugs, particularly cocaine, as a source of false fulfillment for this void. In most cases, cocaine is introduced to an athlete by groupies and friends. It is often used initially to celebrate victory or relieve the agony of defeat. In most cases I have dealt with, cocaine had been used to increase sexual performance.

Few users, however, realize the potential for addiction to cocaine, an addiction that is almost certain in over 50 percent of users and now, with the introduction of smokable cocaine, or crack, possible with only limited use. Of course, cocaine pushers realize this. They also know that top-level athletes are susceptible to cocaine habits and are therefore perfect prey. These athletes are often looking for a release or perhaps an extra boost in competition. They also make enough money to support a serious cocaine habit.

In my early experiences, it was interesting to see drug dealers waiting at airports or outside locker room entrances to actually stuff pouches of cocaine into the gym bags of athletes passing by. Giving an athlete a few grams of coke on the house seemed like an investment to them. Once the pusher hooked a topflight athlete, he (or, in many instances, she) had a prime customer. Even in my experience at the USOC, I witnessed how developing amateurs became easy prey for the dealers. It was good business for the dealer to approach young athletes when they were still on the rise. Once a premier amateur athlete was touted by the media, the dealers would move in.

At the very gates outside the Olympic Training Center in Colorado Springs, athletes were not immune to such advances. Like clockwork, prior to the 1984 and 1988 Olympic Summer Games, drug dealers in expensive cars could be seen lurking outside the Training Center, waiting for the chance to introduce young athletes to cocaine.

One such athlete who allowed cocaine to seriously damage his life and athletic aspirations is Tyrell Biggs, an American boxer who won the gold medal in the super heavyweight division in the 1984 Olympic Games in Los Angeles. I had the opportunity to work with Biggs prior to the '84 Games, after he had been found positive for cocaine use. Realizing that Biggs's cocaine habit (in my opinion, addiction) could cost him his opportunity to compete in the Olympic Games, certain executives from the United States of America Amateur Boxing Federation (USA/ABF) and the USOC set out to put Biggs on a rehabilitation program.

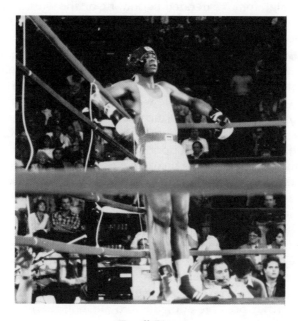

Tyrell Biggs

Indeed, we were able to help Biggs kick his habit (at least temporarily) through the Olympic Games. Once the Games were over, though, Biggs returned to cocaine. I haven't heard from him since. Sources tell me that Biggs's professional career has been all but washed up, thanks to his inability to overcome his cocaine addiction.

Cocaine is a central nervous stimulant. When snorted, cocaine affects the brain within a few minutes, the effects peaking within 15 to 20 minutes and disappearing within an hour. Injected, cocaine takes about 15 seconds to reach the brain, whereas crack, or freebased (smoked), cocaine can begin affecting the body in less than 10 seconds.

Various theories as to how cocaine works have been developed in recent years (see Figure 2). The most popular is that cocaine stimulates neurotransmitters in the brain to increase concentrations of dopamine and norepinephrine, which are naturally secreted chemicals that stimulate brain activity. This action is also typical of amphetamines and amphetamine derivatives, but cocaine also blocks the reabsorption of these transmitters. Most of the effect of this process is mediated through the mid-inner brain area associated with emotion, the so-called pleasure brain area, which coordinates such functions as changes in mood, sexual drive, memory, arousal, friendliness, elation, and vigor. The rush of self-satisfaction that follows cocaine use unleashes a temporary sense of invincibility, power, and aggressiveness that cannot be controlled by outside influences. These feelings disappear within minutes. For a cocaine user to stay high for an extended period, he or she would have to repeat the process over and over, and so cocaine addiction can be a severe financial drain to the user.

The dangers of cocaine are almost limitless. They certainly overshadow the brief high a user feels. The neurological explosion that follows cocaine ingestion transcends the mid-inner brain area, sending mixed signals to other organ systems. An example would be cocaine's stimulation of the heart rate and blood pressure, which happens so suddenly and strongly that it may cause the heart to work twice as hard as it normally does, without giving it time to warm up.[16] This may lead to heartbeat irregularities that can actually stop the heart and cause cardiac arrest and death. The brain itself can also get so many circuits going at the same time that convulsions or seizures can result, potentially causing death. A combination of these events is probably what killed Len Bias.

Repeated use of cocaine and other stimulants can cause a spectrum of side effects from heart failure to non-life-threatening damage, such as the destruction of nasal cartilage from repeated snorting. Smoking cocaine produces such a powerful effect that the user may feel a need for other drugs to stem the depression and exhaustion that occur after use, thus leading to further possible addictions to alcohol, marijuana, sedatives, and other polypharmacies.

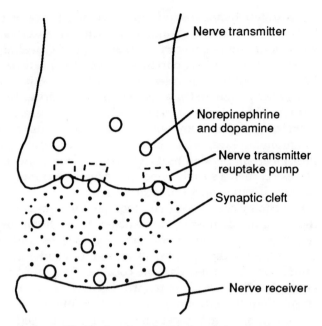

*Normal nerve transmission:*   The molecules of norepinephrine (and dopamine) cross the synaptic cleft to stimulate the receiving nerve cell. Molecules that aren't used are taken up by the nerve transmitter cell.

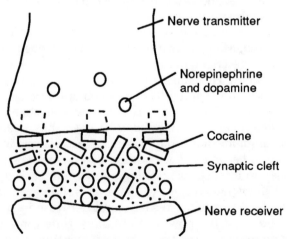

*Cocaine's influence on nerve transmission:*   In the presence of cocaine, the action of the nerve transmitter reuptake pump is blocked so the number of molecules of norepinephrine increases in the synaptic cleft, making the action maximum and prolonged.

**Figure 2.**   How cocaine functions.

An athlete I once treated repeatedly used cocaine to get high for 16 to 24 hours to get him through a competition. Afterwards he would be so strung out and feel so terrible that he used Quaaludes (methaqualone), or, in the black market parlance, ludes, to come down or help him sleep. When he couldn't get ludes, he would use marijuana or just put himself away with booze. In the armamentarium of drugs he carried were ludes; glutethimide (Doriden), which he sometimes dissolved in cough syrups containing codeine, known as syrup and beans; and speed drugs such as amphetamines, which came in different forms called Black Beauties, Pink Hearts, Speckled Birds, Christmas Trees, and various other names. He also carried a supply of benzodiazepines, tranquilizers that he labeled Roches, Tranks, and Pumpkin Seeds.

Personality changes are common among stimulant users, often making them paranoid, hostile, and subject to irrational behavior. More than 50 percent of users lose family, friends, spouses, and careers at some point during their addictions. We often hear of incidents where persons steal, injure, or kill while high on cocaine. One out of every four addicts attempts suicide at some point.[17] Because cocaine is so highly addictive and the euphoric feelings produced so intense, a user sometimes does just about anything to get one more fix. The need to stay high requires large amounts of money to support a habit. Thus, users usually end up selling everything to buy cocaine. When off the drug, the user may become irrational, a volatile time bomb waiting to explode. Also, because this is a short-acting drug, the cycle repeats itself, over and over, more viciously with every turn.

Ingenious methods to get money are found by users desperate to buy more cocaine. Many an institution has been robbed for this purpose. An athlete once described to me how he was able to finance his cocaine habit for just 1 month. He left his expensive car parked on a ghetto street known for crime activity. There it was stripped and trashed overnight. He collected insurance on the basis that his car was stolen and never found.

The cheapness and availability of crack has made cocaine use the national epidemic it is today. Users have explained to me that it doesn't take long to become a crack addict. When crack is smoked, the user experiences an intense rush lasting a few minutes, followed by a state of lesser excitement. Within 5 to 15 minutes, however, the feeling is gone, replaced by an irritable, restless, and depressed state. Although some users who snort the powder form often glide through this period, the downside for crack users is so intense that they almost immediately try to repeat the experience. Both infrequent and long-term users turn to other drugs such as alcohol, marijuana, or even heroin to extend the high period or cushion the resulting crash if they can't get more cocaine.

Addiction to crack has been shown to result from as little as two uses. Now, if we think most people are willing to try anything once or twice, is it any wonder many experts are saying our whole society may be at risk?

## Sympathomimetic Amines

A less dangerous but equally important group of stimulant drugs abused by athletes are the sympathomimetic amines, particularly ephedrine and its derivatives. Ephedrine, pseudoephedrine, phenylpropanolamine, and phenylephrine are stimulants found in some over-the-counter cough, cold, and sinus medications. Because these medicines, widely used by society, are so readily available, they are easily abused by competing athletes for their stimulant effects.

The IOC and the USOC consider sympathomimetic amines banned substances because they can be used for their stimulant effect, though they are also commonly sought for their intended uses. Athletes can get caught up in the innocent or inadvertent use of these drugs during or before competition, and testing may find them positive for a doping violation. As little as one dose of a sympathomimetic amine can cause an athlete to be disqualified for doping. This has been a source of controversy and concern among drug testing officials worldwide.

---

*Author's Note:*   In 1990 the NCAA dropped this category of drugs from the list of substances athletes will be tested for. I think that was a poor decision. Cheaters know they can now use ephedrine to get just as hyped as they possibly can.

---

One might recall the case of Rick DeMont, the American swimmer who was stripped of his gold medal in the men's 400-meter freestyle after testing positive for ephedrine at the 1972 Olympic Games in Munich. DeMont claimed the drug in his system was a by-product of asthma medication (Marax) he had been given by his physician before departing for the Olympic Games. Indeed, he probably used this medication solely to treat his asthma, not to gain some competitive edge in the pool.

The fact remains, though, that DeMont did have the drug in his system at the time of his race. Intentional or not, using this drug may have made DeMont a faster swimmer than he would have been without it. The IOC concluded, therefore, that he had competed under the influence of a performance enhancing drug that may have given him an unfair advantage over his competition. Unfortunately, the IOC had no alternative but to disqualify him for a doping violation. DeMont was subsequently barred from competing in the 1500 freestyle—an event he held the world record in. And that, in my opinion, was unfair, given the circumstances.

Today, declaration of the use of these substances at testing, and quantitative analysis of the amount found in a positive urine test, can constitute grounds for an appeal in the USOC drug testing protocol. Because it is impossible to distinguish the intent of use after an athlete has tested positive, the quantitative amount is determined and compared with the declaration made by the athlete at testing. If the amount is consistent with the declaration, the athlete may receive an acceptance of the appeal. The excuse of inadvertent use, however, is acceptable only one time. The athlete must not make the mistake again.

---

*Author's Note:* Methods adopted by the USOC to prevent innocent or inadvertent use is the subject of a subsequent chapter that will explain how even well-intentioned rules to protect drug-free competitors some-times wind up allowing new ways to beat the drug control system.

---

To avoid this mess, constant education is extremely necessary. Athletes, coaches, trainers, parents, and particularly physicians must be completely aware of the risks these drugs pose to the athlete about to be subjected to drug testing. A physician or parent advising an athlete must continuously remind the athlete of the necessary precautions when using over-the-counter medications.

Generally, these substances clear the system in 48 to 72 hours, giving athletes ample time to stop use before competition. There are also acceptable alternative decongestants, such as oxymetazoline, found in over-the-counter nasal sprays such as Afrin, Otrivin, and Sine-Aid, which are not banned and can be substituted for the banned decongestants.

As in most cases, athletes are fully aware of the options available to them to beat the system. Because of these loopholes, stimulant use still remains popular to a certain extent, despite the fact that we are able to effectively combat stimulant use with postcompetition testing.

Stimulants were first widely used in the sport of cycling. Cyclists have a long, notorious history of drug use. I have already described how stimulant use has been commonplace in cycling since the mid- to late 19th century. Today, however, the U.S. Cycling Federation is, in my opinion, among the most progressive sport federations when it comes to testing and trying to stop drug abuse at the amateur level. U.S. Cycling Federation Executive Director Jerry Lace is one of the most effective leaders on this front.

Stimulant use, however, is still relatively common among professional cyclists. Jeannie Longo of France, the former world champion professional female cyclist, and a three-time winner of the Tour de France Feminins, publicly refused to come to the United States for competitions as long as I was the director of Sports Medicine and Science at the USOC.

Longo had competed in the United States frequently before 1986. During the World Championships of Cycling in Colorado Springs in November of 1986, she attempted to break the world record for 3 kilometers. Indeed, her time was quick enough to break American Rebecca Twigg's world record. However, I was then in charge of overseeing drug testing for the

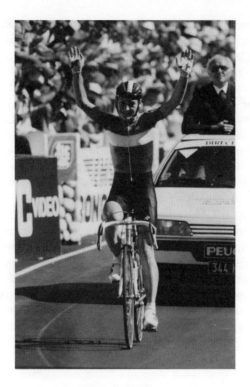

Jeannie Longo
*Note.* Photograph reprinted by permission of AP/Wide World Photos.

U.S. Cycling Federation. After Longo broke the record, a postcompetition drug test revealed significant traces of ephedrine, a central nervous system stimulant, in Longo's urine.

Of course, Longo vehemently denied using any drugs, claiming that I was trying to undermine her for whatever ill-conceived reason. But the evidence was conclusive, and the results were reported to the international cycling union (the Federation International Amateur de Cyclisme) and Longo's national cycling body. Her 3-kilometer record was disallowed.

In the following month, Longo went on to set world marks in the 5K, the 10K, and the 1-hour distance events. She returned to France and pleaded her case before the French cycling officials, who, after being pressured by an angry Federation International Amateur de Cyclisme, reluctantly upheld the decision to disallow her 3K world record but allowed the other three records to stand. I think at least a long suspension would have been in order, but cycling policies only allow for a 30-day suspension, a slap on the wrist and a weak signal to young riders regarding the use of stimulants. Needless to say, Longo was stung by the exposé, but she was ultimately able to beat the system (at least partially) and complain to the world that drug testing in the United States was unfair.

This situation has since generated much discussion among drug testing officials worldwide. Evidently, Longo had tested positive for stimulants before the incident in Colorado Springs, and I understand that she has even been found positive in the very recent past. I received, from a very reliable confidential source, confirmation that in 1986 Longo was taking a French product called Exosuline, which contains 25 mg of ephedrine (a sympathomimetic amine) per capsule. In fact, Longo had actually admitted off the record to using this drug earlier that year. I received the actual product from France, analyzed it, and was able to confirm without a doubt that indeed this was the product Longo was using to enhance her performance in Colorado Springs.

I never understood why she singled me or the United States out for criticism, other than the fact that testing in France and elsewhere in Europe was not as sophisticated as in the United States. Hence, she couldn't pass the drug tests as easily in this country. I guess our feelings about one another are somewhat mutual, although to me this isn't a personal matter, it is a matter of fair competition and maintaining legitimate world records. By the way, Longo did eventually break Twigg's 3K record in Mexico City in September 1989.

### Caffeine

Caffeine, one of the world's most popular drugs, is also a central nervous system stimulant used by athletes to get that little extra boost before competing. Caffeine can be found in coffee, tea, cocoa, and a host of other products, including diet pills and cold medicines.

The effects of the drug depend heavily on the amount an individual consumes: the larger the dose, the greater the stimulant effect. The average amount of caffeine in a cup of brewed coffee is approximately 100 to 150 mg, whereas a cup of instant coffee may contain from 80 to 100 mg or less. To the surprise of many, a single cup of tea can contain anywhere from 30 to 75 mg of caffeine. Cola drinks contain an average of 35 mg of caffeine per 12-ounce can.

When a person drinks a cup of coffee, the effects of caffeine begin within 20 minutes. The drinker's metabolism, body temperature, and blood pressure all increase. Caffeine also has a diuretic effect (increasing urine production), which can lead to dehydration. Other detrimental side effects include elevated blood sugar levels, hand tremors, decreased appetite, and delayed sleep. Extremely high levels of caffeine in the system can cause nausea, diarrhea, trembling, headache, and nervousness.[18]

Despite the potential pitfalls an athlete may encounter by taking caffeine, this drug became popular in sports after certain scientific studies showed caffeine's ability to burn blood fats for energy. The thought here is that endurance may increase by cranking in with the fatty acid cycle of metabolism before utilizing normal stored energy sources.

This notion is still somewhat controversial, but word of performance enhancement spreads like wildfire and sticks like flypaper in the sports community. As with most performance enhancing substances, it doesn't matter whether the substance is scientifically proven to be effective. If athletes perceive benefit from its use, that's all that's necessary for them to continue using it. Caffeine use is probably most popular among runners and cyclists, who use this drug hoping to increase the effects of maximal oxygen consumption and endurance.

The dehydration and fatigue brought on by caffeine use, however, may ultimately negate any advantage this drug might offer. Caffeine also contributes to inflammation of fibromuscular tissue (fibromyositis). This condition, common among athletes, can actually contribute to muscle weakness and tendinitis.

Like ephedrine and its derivatives, caffeine is a difficult drug to ban and control because it is so readily available and widely consumed by the general public. Therefore, a threshold for illegal urine level of caffeine in athletes has been set by the IOC Medical Commission, initially 15 micrograms per milliliter (mcg/ml)—well above the level considered to be an abnormal concentration in the body. This threshold was chosen to make sure no one was unfairly penalized for moderate use but supposedly low enough to catch those using caffeine to cheat. In 1987 the level was dropped to 12 mcg/ml.

To reach a level of 12 mcg/ml of caffeine in the urine, however, an athlete would have to drink, within minutes of competition, approximately 8 cups of standard American brewed coffee (each cup containing 150 mg of caffeine, equivalent to 1.5 mcg per serving; 1.5 mcg × 8 cups equals a level of 12 mcg/ml 2 to 3 hours after use). You get the picture of just how high these standards actually are.

To ingest this much caffeine at one time would probably cause more harm than good, considering that caffeine is a gastric irritant that can cause stomach cramps and diarrhea—not what someone would like to experience in a road race.

Believe it or not, athletes have even found ways to circumvent this problem. Some use caffeine in an enema or in little pink suppositories, which I intercepted from members of the United States Cycling Team during the 1984 Olympic Games. Each of these suppositories contained the caffeine equivalent of 25 cups of coffee. This was, to the cyclists, a smart idea. The suppository method bypassed the stomach by putting the drug in the other end of the gastrointestinal tract, thus avoiding most of the irritation.

Believe me when I say athletes and their advisory gurus go to any length and often find ingenious methods to gain some competitive edge. A cyclist in the 1988 United States Olympic Trials was found positive for caffeine and admitted that he had injected caffeine directly into his bloodstream. In other words, he was mainlining caffeine. It's hard to imagine where all this will end.

## NARCOTICS

Opium, derived from the poppy plant, is one of the oldest drugs known. Narcotics are the derivatives of opium, namely, morphine, codeine, and other drugs used to counter pain and create hallucinatory, euphoric effects. The addictive nature of narcotics is well known. Their ability to help the body perform are not well accepted; therefore, one cannot argue that these drugs should be banned on the basis that they enhance performance. The abuse of narcotics among athletes seems to be more directly related to these drugs' effectiveness in allaying pain. Narcotics *are*, therefore, banned substances.

Because the pressure on athletes to perform well is so intense, they sometimes turn to narcotics as an emotional escape. As with cocaine, this can lead to deadly addiction. The pain blocking effects of narcotics can sometimes fool an athlete into attempting feats he or she may be physically incapable of accomplishing by normal means. When the body signals pain to the brain, it is for a reason; when the mind is under the influence of narcotics, it can't always read body signals correctly. This, understandably, could lead to serious injuries. For example, it is possible for weight lifters to rupture muscles by attempting weights that far exceed their normal lift capacities, if they shoot themselves up with enough narcotics before their attempts.

By banning these drugs, we are able to limit the potential abuses that may lead to career ending injuries as well as to reduce the risk for tragic addictions. The death of Baltimore Colts great "Big Daddy" Lipscomb, caused by heroin addiction in 1963, still serves as one of the most infamous examples of a narcotic-related tragedy.

Fortunately, the IOC has also banned the use of local anesthetics as pain-killers in sport. I firmly believe the now common use of anti-inflammatory drugs such as ibuprofen, Naprosyn, Indocin, and yes, even aspirin, should be banned if the IOC and the USOC are to prevent performance enhancement through reduction of pain. Also, banning aspirin and other anti-inflammatory drugs would be effective in preventing unnecessary bleeding, particularly in contact sports.

## BETA-BLOCKERS

Beta-adrenergic blockers are banned in general—along with sedatives, hypnotics, tranquilizers, antidepressants, anticonvulsants, and alcohol—

## BANNED NARCOTIC ANALGESICS

| Generic name | Example |
|---|---|
| Alphaprodine | Nisentil |
| Anileridine | Leritine, Apodol |
| Buprenorphine | Buprenex |
| Codeine | Codicept (Germany), Codipertussin (Germany) |
| Dextromoramide | Palfium, Jetrium, Narcolo |
| Dextropropoxyphene | Darvon |
| Diamorphine | Heroin |
| Dihydrocodeine | Synalogos DC, Paracodin |
| Dipipanone | Diconal, Wellconal |
| Ethoheptazine | Panalgin (Italy), Equagesic |
| Ethylmorphine | Diosan comp (Spain), Trachyl (France) |
| Levorphanol | Levo-Dromoran |
| Methadone HCl | Dolophine, Amidone |
| Morphine | Cyclimorph 10, Durmorph, MS Continus |
| Nalbuphine | Nubain |
| Pentazocine | Talwin |
| Pethidine | Demerol, Centralgin, Dolantin, Dolosal, Pethold |
| Phenazocine | Narphen |
| Trimeperidine | Demerol, Mepergan |

### . . . and related compounds, e.g.:

| | |
|---|---|
| Hydrocodone | Hycodan, Tussionex, Vicodin |
| Oxomorphine | Narcan |
| Oxycodone | Percodan |
| Hydromorphone | Dilaudid |
| Tincture of opium | Paregoric |

From: U.S. Olympic Committee drug education handbook *Drug Free*, 1989-1992.

for certain sports such as shooting, biathlon, and modern pentathlon. Clinically, these drugs are used to prevent migraines and cardiac arrhythmias and treat hypertension, anxiety, and certain movement tremors.

Some athletes use these drugs to calm anxiety and nervous tension in sports where physical activity is not stressed. Marksmen, golfers, archers, and trapshooters have used beta-blockers to achieve steadiness of the hands, particularly the trigger finger, and to assist sleep and rest before competitions. Because beta-blockers can slow the heart rate, skiers and

## BANNED BETA-BLOCKERS

| Generic name | Example |
| --- | --- |
| Acebutolol | Sectral |
| Alprenolol | Aptine (France), Betacard (Australia), Sinalol (Japan) |
| Atenolol | Tenormin |
| Labetalol | Normodyne, Trandate |
| Metoprolol | Lopressor |
| Nadolol | Corgard |
| Oxprenolol | Apsolox, Oxanol (Spain), Trasacor (Japan) |
| Pindolol | Visken |
| Propranolol | Inderal |
| Sotalol | Beta-cardone (Argentina), Sotalex (Germany) |
| Timolol | Blocadren |

**. . . and related compounds.**

From: U.S. Olympic Committee drug education handbook *Drug Free*, 1989-1992.

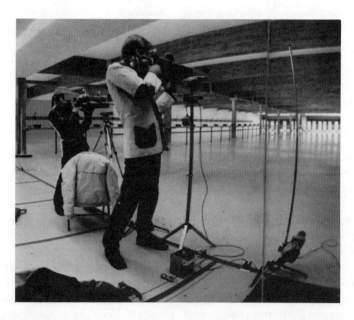

Beta-blockers help steady the trigger fingers of shooters by slowing the heart rate.

ski jumpers have used beta-blockers to help decrease palpitations before their runs. Also, figure skaters—who must perform school figures, a nerve-wracking performance that is part of the overall competition—have used tranquilizers and beta-blocker drugs to steady their motions.

Probably the most dramatic example of performance enhancement through chemistry is the use of beta-blocker drugs in shooting sports. I learned a great deal about this from modern pentathlon athletes. They told me they could take two to three times the normal therapeutic dose of, for example, propranolol (Inderal), a beta-blocker commonly used to reduce blood pressure and slow the heart rate. They could thus decrease the intention tremor and fine movements of their hands and trigger fingers. With heart rates slowed to about 30 beats per minute (or 1 heart-beat every 2 seconds), they could actually pull the trigger between 2 beats of the heart. Thus, their scores far exceeded anything they could do naturally.

## DIURETICS

The newest category added to the banned substance list is diuretics. It was added in April of 1986 and was first considered a member of the doping class at the 1988 Olympic Games. Diuretics do have important therapeutic applications: They are used to treat high blood pressure and problems in fluid retention. Unfortunately, many athletes use these drugs to lose weight in order to meet weight limitations in such sports as wrestling, boxing, judo, and weight lifting. In addition, diuretics are used illegally to escape detection of banned substances by diluting the urine.

Diuretics alter the balance between electrolytes and fluids, causing weight loss by dehydrating fat, which is 70 percent water. This is perceived as fat loss by the athletes. Anabolic-androgenic steroid users also use diuretics to rid their bodies of extra fluid buildup.

Significant diuretic-induced weight (water) loss (greater than 3 percent of body weight) in 24 hours may cause leg and stomach muscle cramps. Diuretics may also hamper the body's ability to regulate its temperature, leading to exhaustion, altered electrolyte balance, cardiac arrhythmia, and ultimately cardiac arrest and death. In 1980 the International Federation of Body Builders (IFBB) Mr. Universe died of a heart attack caused by diuretic use. Weeks later, a Swedish body builder died from complications also caused by diuretic use.

The IOC, as documented in their antidoping charter, believes that "deliberate attempts to reduce weight artificially in order to compete in lower weight classes or to dilute urine constitute clear manipulations which are unacceptable on ethical grounds." Athletes need to receive more education in appropriate weight management and fluid balance by

---

### BANNED DIURETICS

| Generic name | Example |
| --- | --- |
| Acetazolamide | Diamox, AK-Zol, Dazamide |
| Amiloride | Midamor |
| Bendroflumethiazide | Naturetin |
| Benzthiazide | Aquatag, Exna, Hydrew, Marazide, Proaqua |
| Bumetanide | Bumex |
| Canrenone | Aldactone (Germany), Phanurane (France), Soldactone (Switzerland) |
| Chlormerodrin | Orimercur (Spain) |
| Chlorthalidone | Hygroton, Hylidone, Thalitone |
| Diclofenamide | Daranide |
| Ethacrynic acid | Edecrin |
| Furosemide | Lasix |
| Hydrochlorothiazide | Esidrix, HydroDIURIL, Oretic, Thiuretic |
| Mersalyl | Mersalyl Injection |
| Spironolactone | Alatone, Aldactone |
| Triamterene | Dyrenium, Dyazide |

### . . . and related compounds.

From: U.S. Olympic Committee drug education handbook *Drug Free*, 1989-1992.

---

their team physicians. Rapid weight loss over 24 to 48 hours can only be attributed to water loss, which can only lead to easy fatigability, muscle weakness, and cramps. Athletes with persistent problems in making weight need to be encouraged to move up to the next weight class.

Sadly, we don't really know to what extent the drug gurus can go to find new methods of cheating. Even some well-meaning parents can be caught up in this business of doping. I once received a call on the drug hotline from the father of an aspiring national swimmer on the women's team. His daughter's generous breasts were creating an obvious drag and preventing her times from improving. He thought I could recommend a so-called brake drug to slow down her hormonal changes and retard her sexual maturation and adulthood. He didn't ask about the negative effects brake drugs could have on his daughter's body. Amazingly, this father was a physician!

It's safe to say that doping control officials have the upper hand today when it comes to curtailing stimulant, narcotic, beta-blocker, and diuretic use among athletes. However, such use constitutes just a few facets of the drug issue. In athletes' attempts to be swifter, be stronger, and soar higher, they have found other drugs that can get the job done with great effectiveness, drugs that are just as deadly and extremely difficult to detect.

# 4

# Vogue

## Growth Hormone, Blood Doping, and Erythropoietin

One only has to work in the inner circle of amateur sports to fully realize how ingenious and innovative athletes are when it comes to the science of performance enhancement. There's little doubt in my mind that athletes will remain years ahead of the drug testing initiative when it comes to anabolic-androgenic steroids so long as the sport-governing bodies are not willing to commit themselves financially to solving the problem.

Most athletes know how to discontinue drug use in time to avoid detection. We're also beginning to understand that athletes have two other extremely effective cheating methods they can use to gain a competitive edge, methods that are totally undetectable by most present doping control laboratory technology. These methods are the use of growth hormone (GH) and blood doping.

### GROWTH HORMONE

Use of GH, like use of all drugs in sport, is not a new phenomenon. Terry Todd, a former champion power lifter and now professor of kinesiology at the University of Texas, was one of the first to bring this topic to light when he sounded the alarm that human growth hormone was being widely used by college football players in the early 1980s.

Human growth hormone (hGH) is a powerful anabolic hormone that is naturally produced and secreted by the human pituitary gland to regulate growth and development. A lack of naturally produced growth hormone causes the condition of dwarfism, where the individual never reaches full body development. Those suffering from natural growth hormone deficiency, however, can be treated with growth hormone supplementation. For years this has been done by injecting patients with real human growth hormone (which is isolated from the pituitary gland of cadavers).

Prior to 1986 cadavers were the only source of growth hormone. Because growth hormone had to be harvested from the pituitary glands of cadavers, a very limited supply of the drug existed throughout the world. In addition, the cost for natural cadaver-extracted hormone was very, very high—often between $200 and $1000 for a 1-month supply. To make matters worse, much of the GH available to children with growth deficiency was used up by the athletic black market.

Price to the athlete was often quite irrelevant, so not many were turned off by the high cost of growth hormone. In 1984, however, several cases of death from a latent viral disease called Creutzfeldt-Jakob were attributed to human growth hormone. News of this disease, a fatal neurological disorder that takes years to incubate (like the AIDS virus), quickly halted sales. Anyone who had used hGH in the past 10 years was susceptible to contracting the disease. Human growth hormone was promptly removed from the legitimate American pharmaceutical market.

This solved the problem of abuse by athletes for a short period of time. Unbelievably, but true, the drug gurus, undaunted, began selling monkey (simian and rhesus) and cow (bovine) growth hormone to athletes.

I doubt that bovine GH ever worked in humans, but monkey GH may be a different story. In April 1987 Robert B. Kerr, MD, of San Gabriel, California (considered by many to be one of the world's steroid experts), stated before a congressional committee that he observed significant body changes in persons who used monkey GH. Athletes have told me that monkey GH causes more body hair growth.

Observations such as these may seem absurd, for there is documented evidence that GH is species specific. Unfortunately, our medical research community is once again tardy in settling this question—it might even be altogether disinterested. So a lot of innocent, unsuspecting athletes are taking considerable risks and paying out a fortune in money to learn the hard way.

The problem of growth hormone use is quite complex. There are two things about GH that athletes believe to be true. First, growth hormone works as an anabolic agent to build muscle mass. Whether growth hormone increases strength and whether it is capable of increasing, say, thigh muscle by 2 inches in 1 year are the subjects of heated debate. Whether GH actually works, however, doesn't really matter: The athlete who thinks it works will use it.

Second, growth hormone cannot be detected by any drug test presently used to control doping in international competition. It is possible for an athlete to use growth hormone and still pass all after-competition drug tests.

Athletes using growth hormone think that this drug can increase their muscle size, their bone growth, and the strength of connective tissues in their bodies, thus giving them an added power advantage on the playing field. In certain respects, however, such growth can cause some of the major problems associated with GH use. Every part of the body grows. That can cause a lot of problems. In addition, athletes claim they don't feel as good when they use GH as they feel when using AAS.

Some researchers have suggested that growth hormone is not as effective in building muscle as are anabolic-androgenic steroids. Others, however, feel that when growth hormone is used with AAS or testosterone, the anabolic effects of these latter drugs can be compounded. Athletes also feel that tendon and ligament problems (tendinitis and ligament ruptures) commonly associated with anabolic-androgenic steroid use don't occur when growth hormone is added to the cycle.

Anabolic-androgenic steroids specifically enlarge only muscle. Growth hormone, on the other hand, stimulates the growth of all tissues, including internal organs. This can lead to a variety of complications, such as enlargement of the spleen and of the liver. This, in turn, could create fatalities in contact sports.

Hypertrophy (expansion) may also occur in the skin, the tongue, and the bones. GH can cause enlargement of facial features, including nose, ears, and tongue—complications commonly seen in the medical syndrome called acromegaly. With this condition, the soft tissues of the hands, feet, jaw, and forehead become overdeveloped, resulting in an enlarged nose, fingers, ears, and toes. This gives one the appearance of the professional wrestler Andre the Giant, who is believed to have been affected by a natural pituitary abnormality.

Growth hormone also decreases the layer of protective fat that surrounds abdominal organs, making GH use an even greater risk in contact sports.

Perhaps as many as 80 percent of growth hormone users develop diabetes requiring insulin treatment. Thyroid disease, menstrual disorders, decrease in sexual drive, and impotence have also resulted from GH use. Many researchers believe that growth hormone use also significantly shortens the user's lifespan.

Athletes don't seem to be phased by these potential problems. In fact, growth hormone seems to remain extremely popular. One of the most terrifying excerpts from *The Underground Steroid User's Handbook* describes growth hormone as follows:

> Wow, is this great stuff! It is the best drug for permanent muscle gains. It is the basic pituitary hormone that makes your

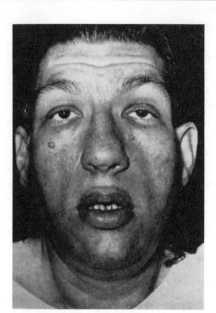

Note the enlarged nose, lips, and jaw of this acromegalic.
*Note.* From *Physical Diagnosis: The History and Examination of the Patient* (p. 57) by J.A. Prior and J.S. Silberstein, 1969, St. Louis: Mosby. Copyright 1969. Reprinted by permission.

whole body grow. People who use it can expect to gain 30 to 40 lbs. of muscle in ten weeks if they can eat about 10,000 calories per day. It is about $600-$800 per 4 vials, and we think this to be another best buy. . . . This is the only drug that can remedy bad genetics as it will make anybody grow. A few side effects can occur, however. It may elongate your chin, feet and hands, but this is arrested with cessation of the drug. Diabetes in teenagers is possible with it. It can also thicken your rib-cage and wrists. Massive increases in weight over such a short time can, of course, give you heart problems. We have heard of a powerlifter getting a heart attack while on GH. GH use is the biggest gamble an athlete can take, as the side effects are irreversible. Even with all that, we LOVE the stuff.

Can you believe this? This kind of underground "education" is, in my mind, criminal. If it came from a physician, it would be considered malpractice. Why won't physicians counter this lunacy? I guess that's why I keep writing.

The problems associated with growth hormone become significantly more dangerous when you consider that an overzealous parent, impatient with a child's growth and development, might begin the kid on a program of growth hormone. Say, for example, a 13-year-old child at 100 pounds isn't big enough to make an impact on the local peewee football team. It could be very easy, in our society, for a father to convince himself, or even his doctor, to give the boy growth hormone to bring him up in size. Can you, though, imagine yourself as a parent making this kind of judgment, fooling with Mother Nature?

Growth hormone should be used only on children who a medical doctor has diagnosed as growth hormone deficient, and used only under the physician's care. I urge all parents to let their children's bodies take their natural courses. It is not right for a parent to decide to give a child a dangerous drug for the sole purpose of enhancing athletic ability. Growth hormone can have profound and even life-threatening effects. To give this drug to an otherwise normal boy or girl is *wrong*.

Unfortunately, it seems like there are, and always will be, some individuals impatient or foolish enough to take chances with GH, particularly when the potential for high school popularity, college scholarships, and even multimillion-dollar professional contracts hang in the balance.

William Taylor, MD, another pioneer in alerting the medical profession and public to the abuse of anabolic-androgenic steroids in sport, also warned athletes about the dangers of GH use in his book *Hormonal Manipulation: A New Era of Monstrous Athletes*. Dr. Taylor's attempts to warn the medical profession of GH problems went unheeded (like the attempts of most pioneers in recognizing abuse). Nonetheless, he introduced to the world of sport the prospect of "a new era of monstrous athletes." He related the known use of growth hormone as early as 1981.

Dr. Kerr reported in a 1985 edition of the *New Zealand Journal of Sports Medicine* that growth hormone "is the elite drug in track and field competition today . . . all over the world."[19]

Thanks to our pharmaceutical industry, many of the problems associated with human GH (hGH) were solved with the 1986 advent of recombinant DNA synthesized GH. This has made GH not only more available but also cheaper.

Recent discussions I've had with athletes indicate that synthetic growth hormone is not as effective as the real thing. So, when they can get hGH, athletes jump at the opportunity, despite the risk of contracting diseases. That's why there is still a market for hGH.

Today synthetic growth hormone is readily available to athletes, in spite of claims by the country's two producers of synthetic growth hormone—Eli Lilly and Genentech—that they tightly control all sales. Is there a need for better control? I think so. Athletes tell me it is not a problem to buy synthetic GH.

In recent black market order forms, I have even noticed the continued availability of human growth hormone. Obviously, hGH is still produced overseas because none is currently being produced in the United States.

Two foreign labs, to my knowledge, still produce human growth hormone. They are Serano Labs, which produces Assellacrin, and Pharmacia Labs, Inc., which produces Crescormon.

I find it hard to believe that hGH is still being marketed at all, especially in view of the potential for latent virus diseases, including AIDS, that can be found in human tissue. It might be that the black marketeers are just using up old supplies of Assellacrin and Crescormon. Then again, I also wonder how much of the black market hGH is the real thing. One cannot really trust the black market. After all, there is no honor among thieves. I have investigated at least one vial of Crescormon, which was given to me by a suspicious athlete who wasn't realizing the effects he was hoping for. Indeed, I discovered that he hadn't really gotten hGH, but aqueous testosterone. The product was obviously counterfeit, which is not surprising when one considers the profit motives of the crooks who sell illegitimate drugs. The athlete in question paid $450 and got $15 worth of aqueous testosterone.

---

*Author's Note:*   I can't stress enough to the athlete contemplating purchasing illegitimate drugs the old axiom "Let the buyer beware."

---

Media attention recently focused on the use of growth hormone when Darrell Robinson, the 1986 American 400-meter dash champion, accused 1988 Olympic women's sprint champion Florence Griffith Joyner of purchasing human growth hormone from him to help her prepare for the 1988 Olympic Trials and the Olympic Games in Seoul. Robinson stated that Griffith Joyner gave him $2,000 for a 10-cc vial of human growth hormone. Robinson's accusations were first published in a 1989 issue of the West German magazine *Stern* (Robinson was reportedly paid $50,000 for the story). Days later both athletes appeared on NBC's *Today* show, where Griffith Joyner discredited Robinson's story, calling him a "compulsive, crazy, lying lunatic."

The question of whether Florence Griffith Joyner (Flo Jo) used performance enhancing substances to help her reach her Olympic goals may never be fully resolved. All I can say is Griffith Joyner was tested at the 1988 Olympic Trials and the Olympic Games. On both occasions, her test results came up negative. Therefore, there isn't one iota of medical proof that would suggest Florence Griffith Joyner competed under the influence of anabolic-androgenic steroids or stimulants.

Unfortunately for Flo Jo, growth hormone use cannot be detected in urine testing; we probably could detect GH use with blood testing, but this is not done at the Olympics. Therefore, she, like many successful, record-breaking athletes, will be painted with the brush of drug-use allegations without a means to protect herself.

There are those who point to Griffith Joyner's incredible muscle development between the 1984 Olympic Games and the 1988 Olympic Games and suggest that this would not be possible for a fully matured athletic female without the use of performance enhancing anabolic agents. A recent secret report out of East Germany (of all places) contended that Griffith Joyner's thigh muscles had expanded by 2 inches in 1 year. According to the medical authors of this report, such muscle development is possible "only with a helping substance." In an April 1989 U.S. Senate hearing on the topic of drug abuse in sport, Senator Joseph Biden of Delaware was shown two pictures of Griffith Joyner: one from 1984 and a more recent shot. His remark: "This is two different people."

I'm afraid, however, that these unscientific allegations are extremely unfair, even if possibly true. It's an accusation of guilt without proof and unconstitutional with regard to our principle of "innocent until proven guilty." All legal and medical tests vindicate Griffith Joyner of any drug-use charge.

But considering the loopholes that have existed in drug testing procedures for international competition in recent years, the shady history the IAAF and TAC have had with regard to doping control, the recent claim by IOC Medical Commission Chairman Prince de Merode that 50 track-and-field athletes showed evidence of anabolic-androgenic steroid use but tested negative in the Seoul Olympics, and recent admissions of anabolic-androgenic steroid use that have been made by athletes who cleared the tests, such as sprinter Diane Williams, doubts about drug-free athletes will probably never be erased.

This is quite tragic. If Flo Jo did indeed compete clean, which all medical records seem to indicate, then she will continue to be dogged by a black cloud of suspicion for no fair reason whatsoever. Because of the inherent weakness in testing procedures, we suspect that there are athletes who have used banned substances, have won gold medals in the past, and have gotten away with their drug use. Thus, the majority of athletes who have competed clean are unfairly subjected to suspicion.

The only way I think we could clear this problem up would be to have consistent, reliable testing.

I would love to see Griffith Joyner come out of retirement and volunteer for regular blood drug tests throughout her comeback. By training hard and eating well, she could probably post times within range of her 1988 times. In fact, she might even break her world records, only this time she'd have medical certification to guarantee she wasn't using anything artificial to help her. Only if she were to do this would she put all the rumors and innuendoes to bed. Until that happens, nobody can be sure one way or the other.

As with most medical problems, the professional, academic, and administrative communities have taken their own sweet time in recognizing the fact that there is a problem and finding ways to deal with it. Growth hormone is certainly a shining example of this. Only since this escapade involving Griffith Joyner and Robinson has the subject of growth hormone use received the attention it has deserved, despite the fact that growth hormone has been used in sport for years.

On April 8, 1987, Terry Todd, Dr. Taylor, Dr. Kerr, I, and others testified before the Subcommittee on Health and Environment of the U.S. House of Representatives that we wanted growth hormone to be placed in Category II of the Controlled Substances Act because of its frequent misuse in the world of sport. To this date, nothing has resulted from our testimony.

A major reason the subcommittee did not act to place growth hormone on the controlled substances list at that hearing was the resistance received from the two major pharmaceutical companies that produced the new synthetic, DNA-derived forms of the drug: Genentech, the first company to produce synthetic growth hormone when it created Protropin; and Eli Lilly, the second, producing Humatrope. Defining growth hormone under Category II of the Controlled Substances Act would make manufacturers, pharmacists, and physicians verify and maintain records of use of the drug; any misuse of the drug could bring a punitive fine and a possible jail sentence. The companies have argued that such measures are unnecessary because they were already tightly controlling and documenting the distribution of their growth hormone.

We who had seen the abuse of this drug by athletes knew differently, of course. When we were challenged on this GH distribution issue, Dr. Kerr simply pulled out a vial of Protropin and placed it on the table. He had gone out on the black market and purchased this vial for $450 as evidence to the committee that the industry claims of tight controls didn't hold much water. The flustered Genentech representatives at the hearing disputed our claim and went back to research the vial's serial number and their own distribution records. They returned to claim this vial was part of a shipment that had been stolen.

One really has to wonder why so much resistance to controlling synthetic growth hormone distribution has been raised, because the potential legitimate medical use for this drug is for a very limited population of people who suffer from dwarfism, hardly a large enough group to justify the millions of dollars spent in developing the drug. I have the distinct impression from all this that there is a much bigger market on the horizon for GH: the weight reduction market. Once GH becomes better understood and availability, cost, and safety problems are worked out, it will probably be the drug of choice for adult weight loss programs—controlled, I hope, by the medical profession, and not abused.

Incidentally, this hearing also produced a very memorable moment for me. I was asked why athletes use these drugs, regardless of the risks they pose. My answer was rather facetious. I stated that athletes would use *anything* if they thought it would give them the competitive edge. I illustrated this "whatever it takes to win" philosophy by saying that if I put horse manure in capsules to be taken three times a day and told an athlete that these capsules would make him big and strong, even if he knew they were filled with horse manure, he would take them.

The questioning congressman thought I was being flippant and asked me to refrain from such ridiculous comments, particularly before such a prestigious congressional committee. Terry Todd jumped in to defend me. He said not only would he have used those manure pills if he'd had them while he was competing, but he also would have gone out and bought the biggest, meanest, strongest horse he could find so that he could make the pills himself.

The comments are now part of the *Congressional Record*, and rightly so. I think this story drives home the point of just how committed athletes can be to quack pharmacology in their attempts to gain the winning edge.

The wholesale price of 10 cc (about 1 month's worth of treatments) of growth hormone is around $350. The athlete, however, can usually buy growth hormone only at a premium price on the black market (sometimes 5 to 10 times its wholesale value) or from certain physicians willing to sell this substance to athletes.

From my conversations with athletes, I get the impression that there is more GH being used than even I thought. Its popularity seems to be based on the fact that as yet there is not a laboratory test that diagnoses growth hormone use. It didn't take the athletic community long to discover the anabolic effects of growth hormone and to capitalize on the fact that this drug can be used without fear of detection. At least for now, with urine being the substance used in analysis, no athletic doping test detects GH. By using blood, though, which gives a much more complete picture of the chemicals present in a person's body, we could detect not only present but even past use. See how simple it could be if sport officialdom were committed to stopping the problem?

Scientists know very little about the performance enhancing effects of growth hormone. What we do know is that athletes are using it and subjecting themselves to severe risks. Because GH is not detectable by urinalysis, perhaps drug testing has innocently created another monster, just like athletes are now using the more dangerous forms of anabolic-androgenic steroids because these substances can better help them avoid detection. Sometimes the solution to a problem can be worse than the problem itself. At least we must take this possibility into account as we think out solutions.

Ultimately, there seems to be only one solution to this problem: We need to develop an effective way to test for growth hormone use, both past and present, among athletes. That may mean blood analysis testing because a scientist cannot detect growth hormone metabolites in urine but *could* detect an abnormal concentration of this hormone in a blood sample. Once such a test can be developed, it needs to become part of the rules of fair play: If you use, you don't play. Abiding by universal drug testing standards simply must become, in the minds of the athletes, coaches, and officials, just part of the game.

## BLOOD DOPING AND ERYTHROPOIETIN

This brings me to another new, dangerous practice that is as serious a threat as growth hormone to fair play in sport. Blood doping, blood packing, blood boosting, induced erythrocythemia—I like to use the term *doping*. Let's not sophisticate it. It's cheating. The word *doping* implies unfair play, and that is what it is.

Blood doping entails infusing extra blood into the body to increase the amount of red blood cells carrying oxygen to the muscle cells. Blood doping is done in one of two ways. Initial blood doping technique used blood other than the athlete's own. This was called homologous blood doping. This method has fallen into considerable disrepute because of the potential for allergic reactions, hepatitis, and, most importantly, AIDS.

Therefore, the most popular current method is to remove approximately 2 pints of the athlete's own blood (there are 8 pints total in the human body) some 8 to 12 weeks before competition. The blood is frozen and stored in a blood bank. The athlete then continues to train, but having become anemic, having lost 2 pints of blood, he or she must increase intake of food, vitamins, and iron. This increased diet activity usually replenishes the 2 lost pints of blood in 2 to 3 months.

Then, a day or so before the target competition, the 2 pints of previously extracted blood are thawed. If sophisticated techniques are used, the red blood cells that carry the oxygen are separated from the serum. Those red blood cells are then infused back into the athlete's body. This is called autologous blood doping.

The principle in both methods is rather fundamental: By increasing the number of red blood cells capable of carrying oxygen (the real fuel needed for muscles to work), the athlete can increase both endurance and strength. The body burns off oxygen more rapidly during exercise than during rest. The heart beats faster and the athlete breathes harder during exercise because the body is forced to replenish this oxygen supply at a quicker rate. With an increased number of red blood cells transporting oxygen, the system, in theory, becomes more efficient. In turn, the stress on the body is reduced, and the athlete may have a decided advantage over the competition.

To understand this process better, consider the following analogy. Say a construction foreman has been hired to build a small house out of bricks.

He has 10 men laying the bricks for the house. If he wants to have that house built in 1 day, those men would have to work very fast and exert much energy to get the job done. If he had 20 men working, he would be able to build the same house in 1 day, but the stress on the building crew is reduced. Everyone's load would be considerably less, and the crew would be neither as stressed nor as tired as it would have been with just 10 men.

With blood doping, if an athlete increases the amount of red blood cells working to carry the oxygen throughout the body, the whole system will feel less natural stress, thus creating more capacity to expend energy and more endurance.

Actually, the athlete might do just as well by inhaling pure oxygen. However, that method might make it difficult for an athlete to gain an advantage. One would have to strap an oxygen tank on the back, which might make running a marathon or swimming 400 meters most difficult.

Blood doping was not officially considered cheating by the IOC before 1986. However, it was considered dirty pool by the athletic community. Even today, the debate goes on as to whether blood doping should be considered a doping violation equal in magnitude to the use of performance enhancing drugs, particularly when we consider the fact that a blood doping athlete is using his or her own blood. I have argued this point with certain Soviet and East German officials who think that using one's own blood does not constitute doping.

I firmly believe blood doping is cheating. Remember, the USOC defines doping as "the administration of or use by a competing athlete of any substance foreign to the body or any physiological substance taken in abnormal quantity or taken by an abnormal route of entry into the body with the sole intention of increasing in an artificial and unfair manner his/her performance in competition."

The basis for my argument is this key passage. Though the blood may indeed originate in the athlete's own body, I believe this blood is a "foreign" substance when taken moments before competition. The body has adjusted: It doesn't need this blood, nor does it want this blood. Thus, 2 extra pints in the bloodstream constitute an "abnormal quantity." A transfusion is an "abnormal route of entry into the body." Most important, we know athletes are blood doping with the "sole intention" of gaining an "artificial and unfair" competitive edge.

There is ample scientific evidence in the medical literature that this technique can increase endurance by 17 to 30 percent (depending on which study you read). A study out of the University of New Mexico, for example, demonstrated how blood doping could shave 69 seconds off an athlete's time in a 10,000-meter run. That's impressive: approximately a 3-percent improvement on the world-class level!

In my opinion, even though the individual is using a natural substance (in most cases his or her own blood), blood doping really has to be categorized as cheating and can't be considered fair play. To do otherwise would mean allowing blood doping. If blood doping were allowed, in order to assure fairness to all competitors, we would have to see that all competitors were blood doping. Because blood doping is not necessarily free of serious health risks, this practice could never be accepted by ethical medical standards.

There are several very serious potential hazards associated with blood doping. First, the sudden increase in circulating blood increases the total blood volume, thereby increasing the blood pressure and the work load on the heart. An increase in blood pressure and heart work load might easily cause total heart failure. A backup of fluid in the lungs, called pulmonary edema, also might result; this complication is also potentially lethal.

Second, an increase in the number of red blood cells increases the viscosity, or thickness, of the blood. An increase in blood viscosity can easily lead to an increase in the coagulability of the blood, which in turn may lead to blood clotting and possible stroke. These are serious risks. I have personally seen examples of blood clots occurring in athletes whom I suspected of blood doping.

The normal person's heart is used to pumping blood with no greater than a 55-percent concentration of red blood cells. If that concentration is increased, the system clogs up. Remember, blood cells themselves are not liquid, just carried in liquid. A person's heart pumps blood through arteries like a pump pushes water through a garden hose. When someone has an abnormal concentration of red blood cells, the heart feels similar stress that a pump would feel when forced to push cottage cheese through the garden hose. With enough stress, something is bound to give.

In addition, blood doping requires that several persons be involved, that a blood bank be available, that blood be properly handled, and that all the utensils, tubes, and needles be absolutely sterile. We know unsterile intravenous blood transfusions can cause the transmission of infections. Transfusions have always been dangerous even in the best of hands.

Now, with the danger of the life-threatening AIDS infection, transfusions are even more risky. There are already cases of anabolic-androgenic steroid users who have contracted the AIDS virus through sharing needles with other anabolic-androgenic steroid users. Unfortunately, it might not be too long before some athlete contracts AIDS through blood doping.

Here's another thing to consider: What we know about the science of blood doping is based on the fact that performance enhancement comes from using only 2 pints of blood. Those of us who work with athletes and understand their youthful attitude of indestructibility fully know that 2 extra pints will not always be the limit. Even if all the health risks of 2 extra pints were considered minimal (for whatever ill-conceived reason) and blood doping were considered safe and allowed in international competition, would athletes really stop at 2 extra pints? If everyone were gaining the 2-pint advantage, isn't it reasonable to imagine there would be athletes willing to try 3 or 4 extra pints to stay a step ahead of their competition?

Because of my experiences dealing with athletes who use tremendous doses of anabolic-androgenic steroids, I often ask athletes how many aspirins they would use for a headache. In most cases, the athletes said they would use at least *six*, not two, aspirins for the pain. This is an important point. Athletes would not stop at 2 pints of blood when blood doping. Eventually, they would use more and more until we start seeing really serious effects, until someone blows his heart apart or dies from heart failure in front of a live worldwide television audience. Then sport officials will get excited about controlling this dangerous form of cheating.

There is now even more reason for concern on this front. Scientists are now able to use recombinant DNA synthesis to produce erythropoietin (also known as EPO), which is the body's natural hormone that stimulates red blood cell production. This very potent hormone is capable of increasing the red blood cell count by some 25 to 35 percent. The action of this drug also lasts for a long period of time and is dose related. In other words, the body's buildup of red blood cells from an injection or injections can be progressive.

Along with others in this field, I know for a fact that many athletes are using this hormone to pump up their red blood cell supplies. In fact, we've even begun so see an alarming rise in the number of deaths among European cyclists who use erythropoietin. I'm sure it won't be long before a high-profile American athlete kills himself or herself using this hormone.

Believe you me, it is not too late to do something. Tests for blood doping must be found soon, and that might not be a major problem. (However, the U.S. Olympic Foundation *turned down* worthy research on the effects blood doping has on the body, and on clues for detection, in 1985.)

Blood doping has been around in the world of sport for years. It is most popular among cyclists, runners, and Nordic skiers, though I have heard reports that blood doping has taken place in almost every endurance-type sport.

International media suspicion of an athlete's using blood doping to better his performance first came in 1976, when Finnish distance runner Lasse Viren won the Olympic gold medal in the men's 10,000 meters in Montreal. Less than 24 hours later, Viren returned to the track to win the 5,000 meters also, and 24 hours after that, he finished fifth in the marathon! Realizing that blood doping was first researched and experimented with in the Scandinavian countries, the media grilled Viren about the possibility that he had used blood doping to achieve his miracle performances. Viren consistently denied all allegations.

In 1981 Finnish steeplechaser Mikko Ali-Leppilampi admitted to blood doping before the 1972 Olympic Games in Munich, West Germany. Kaarlo Maaninka, also of Finland, admitted in 1983 that blood doping helped him win bronze and silver medals in the 5,000- and 10,000-meter events, respectively, in the 1980 Olympic Summer Games in Moscow.

Yet, blood doping first gained huge international attention in 1984. The story is one of the darkest episodes in U.S. Olympic history. At the Los Angeles Olympic Summer Games, eight members of the United States Cycling Team—including the 4000-meter individual pursuit gold medalist, Steve Hegg, and the former 3000-meter women's world record holder, Rebecca Twigg—blood doped.

As you will remember, at this time blood doping was not considered a violation by the IOC, though most of us involved in sport felt this was indeed cheating. Realizing that the team would not be sanctioned for blood doping, team coach Eddie Borysewicz (who was also the man responsible for giving his cyclists caffeine suppositories) and team manager Eddie Burke arranged to have the team blood doped with the help of a physician, Herman Falsetti, MD, from the University of Iowa.

Thomas B. Dickson, MD, was the team physician assigned to take care of the cycling team at the Games. But Dickson wasn't told of the coach's and athletes' intentions. Dr. Dickson arrived in Los Angeles 2 days prior to the start of the cyling events. He was told to meet the team at a Ramada Inn, near the outskirts of the competition site. When he arrived at the hotel, this was what he told me he found:

> I got my first word that they were blood doping when I got to the hotel, I think I was walking down the hallway to the room. When I opened the door, there were two people on the beds. Dr. Falsetti was in the room, too.
>
> What they were doing was using the blood of relatives, or people who had the same blood types as the cyclists. A "donor" was put on one bed, where he had a needle stuck in his arm, and a tube that led down to a transfusion bag on the floor. Gravity would take the blood out of their arm and fill the bag.
>
> Then, they had a messenger (whose qualification, interestingly, was that he owned a bike shop in Tijuana) run these blood bags to a local hospital, where they were screened for blood type, etc.
>
> Once the blood came back, it was transfused into the athlete. They did this by rolling one of those portable coat racks between the beds in the room. And they hung the transfusion bag on this coat rack, so that, again, gravity would lead the blood down the tube and into the arm of the athlete on the bed.

When Dr. Dickson arrived, he was shocked. More than half of the team had already been blood doped. Though the athletes had presumably been told that this was not mandatory, several sprinters were waiting at the door for their transfusions. They didn't realize that blood doping wouldn't give them an advantage until Dr. Dickson told them that the blood doping probably wouldn't help sprinters. Consequently, they left.

Some months later this story broke in, of all places, *Rolling Stone* magazine. How this story broke is an interesting exposé on the politics and manipulation that persist in the world of amateur sport. Dr. Dickson certainly did not intend to blow the whistle on these athletes, but because he was concerned with the potential health risks associated with blood doping, he wrote Dr. Daniel Hanley of the USOC a letter that described what he saw in Los Angeles.

Dr. Dickson had reason to be concerned. When you use someone else's blood, even if the blood is screened and matched for blood type (blood types are A, B, AB, and O) and rh factor (positive and negative), there are still possible complications. For women, a bad transfusion can cause their systems to build blood antibodies, which in turn may complicate childbearing. Expert analyses also indicate that approximately 1 in 10 people who blood dope will experience life-threatening reactions as a result. In numerical terms, because 8 cyclists blood doped, the team was really pushing the odds.

Dr. Dickson wrote about his concerns to follow up on the problem, to see whether we might be able to check the athletes involved to be sure they did not suffer any complications. Unfortunately, Dr. Dickson also happened to send a copy of this letter to Rob Lee, who was then president of the U.S. Cycling Federation. Lee was at that time embroiled in a power struggle with certain other members of his organization, and he decided to rattle cycling's cage as much as he could.

Now, no one has come forward to say exactly how this story leaked to the general public. I know I didn't say anything. However, Dr. Dickson later found out that one of Lee's friends happens to be Jann Wenner, editor of *Rolling Stone*. We suspect the story broke through this route. Then again, it would have become public knowledge sooner or later, because whenever more than one person knows a secret, it isn't really a secret, after all.

As expected, sport officialdom—in this case, the USOC—was unprepared and reluctant to handle this obvious and deplorable case of cheating. After the ball was tossed back and forth between the Cycling Federation and the USOC, the USOC finally accepted responsibility and appointed an investigating committee composed of many Sports Medicine Council physicians. Their recommendation to the USOC basically said to take strong disciplinary action.

Unfortunately, the USOC legal minds, armed with the USOC Constitution, didn't feel it was the USOC's prerogative to do anything. The USOC deferred action to the U.S. Cycling Federation. The Federation leveled draconian sanctions (sure) against the athletes and coach: They all received 30-day suspensions. I wonder if that really struck fear in the hearts of prospective cheaters. Neither the IOC nor the International Federation did much better. No medals were taken away. I wonder how the competitors who were beaten by these athletes at the 1984 Olympic Games feel.

The USOC did try to outlaw blood doping, but enforcing the ban has been most difficult. But it doesn't have to be. If the IOC Medical Commission and the national Olympic Committee want to stop the use of both GH and blood doping, a very easy start would be to require blood testing rather than urinalysis testing. In this day and age, taking a small sample of blood is quick, almost painless, and much more reliable.

There exists enough information on GH in the medical literature to come up with a standard for what is considered the normal growth hormone level in the body. Tests are also available that can measure blood antibodies that develop from the use of synthetic growth hormone. Thus far, though, nobody in sport seems willing to use these tests.

Already various blood screening tests are being perfected to identify blood doping. From what documentation already exists, it would even be possible to set a standard hematocrit, or percentage of red blood cells, allowed for fair play.

To date, however, there is no drug test being used to detect athletes who blood dope. The only real threat to athletes who blood dope are the extenuating circumstances that make this practice difficult to do in secret. The need for some medical professional to withdraw the blood, to freeze it (using a complicated quick-freeze technique, not simply throwing the blood into a refrigerator freezer), and to infuse the blood back into the athlete makes blood doping a rather complicated process. Usually it takes three or more people to perform the blood doping.

Another interesting anecdote from the 1984 Olympic Summer Games in Los Angeles involves Martti Vainio, a distance runner from Finland. Vainio was found positive for anabolic-androgenic steroids by the after-competition testing lab in Los Angeles, but he vehemently denied the charges. Vainio thought there was absolutely no way that he could have tested positive for anabolic-androgenic steroids—that is, until he realized what had *really* happened. Vainio had blood doped to prepare for his event in Los Angeles. Unfortunately, he forgot that when his blood was originally removed and frozen, he was in the middle of a cycle of anabolic-androgenic steroid use. Thus, this blood infused back into his body contained traces of AAS, which were metabolized and picked up by his urine test. Vainio was stripped of the silver medal he won for the 10,000 meter run.

One of the most recent ugly exposés of blood doping involved an American, Nordic combined skier Kerry Lynch. Lynch became the first American athlete to win a medal in the world championships of the Nordic combined event when he won a silver medal in the 1987 Nordic World Championships in Obertsdorf, West Germany. Several months later, however, an internal investigation by the United States Ski Association led Lynch to admit he had engaged in blood doping to prepare for the event. Lynch was stripped of his medal.

Lynch's coach, Doug Peterson, who had arranged the blood doping, and Nordic program director Jim Page, who had authorized and funded the blood doping, were both given a slap on the wrist for their actions. Peterson had his responsibilities within the U.S. Ski Association shifted. Page, by that point, had already been given a position within the USOC.

It is important to note that the Lynch and cycling team stories were the only two cases in sport history where athletes have ever really been stuck to the wall concerning blood doping. Though rumors abound that some Italians, Scandinavians, and particularly Eastern Europeans blood dope (and there is no doubt in my mind that these athletes do), the majority of athletes who have been caught red-handed while blood doping were American. In a sense, the 1984 U.S. Cycling Team and Kerry Lynch are the Ben Johnsons of blood doping.

Believe me, American doping control officials have had this fact put in their faces quite often. Though we might be quick to point fingers at the East Germans and the Soviets, everyone involved can now quickly remind us that the only recorded incidents of blood doping have both involved Americans.

In late 1988 I was involved, on behalf of the USOC, in talks with the European Sports Medicine and Anti-Doping Committees. At that time, we were trying to interest Eastern European countries in a combined effort to develop an international movement against doping in sport. (This, by the way, was the initial groundwork for the present agreement between the national Olympic Committees of the USSR and the United States.) One of the most damning attitudes we were forced to deal with was whether the United States could even be trusted. After all, as Sir Arthur Gold of Great Britain so aptly stated, "the cheaters in international sport seem to be Americans, vis-à-vis the blood doping incidents. Are the Americans' intentions, therefore, sincere?"

In my mind, Gold had reason to doubt our national interest and sincerity with regard to doping. After all, Ben Plucknett, an American discus thrower, had tested positive for anabolic-androgenic steroids in a European track event. Two weeks later Plucknett appeared on the cover of a major American newsmagazine as America's athlete of the year.

It is apparent that we need a lot of cooperative effort to gain the confidence of the rest of the world in trying to stop drug abuse in sport. Quite honestly, I am not convinced that some of the leadership of the USOC appreciates this dilemma or is willing to make a significant commitment to turn the tide. Remember, we can point fingers at other countries all day and not get anywhere. We have a serious problem to deal with right here at home. We just aren't getting the job done.

When nations are asked which country is the bad guy when it comes to doping and cheating in sport, many fingers seem to point in one direction. Not toward Eastern Europe. Not toward the Soviet Union. They point toward the United States of America.

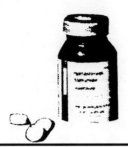

# Drug Testing:
# Foul Play

# 5

# The Counteroffensive

## A New Era of Drug Testing Is Born

Olympic drug testing began in 1968, but before 1983 drug testing and detection at all international competitions was very ineffective, simply because the technology available was primitive and undependable.

As I have described, after-competition testing requires an athlete to submit a urine sample for laboratory analysis immediately after competing. This sample is analyzed in a doping control laboratory by various scientific tests that expose traces of banned substances that have been processed or broken down by the athlete's body and passed into the urine. These by-products are called metabolites.

Before 1983 the technology used in this type of testing was often not sophisticated enough to accurately detect some of the fine metabolites of various stimulants. These tests were certainly ill-equipped to detect the use of anabolic-androgenic steroids with reliable accuracy. Consequently, many athletes were able to clear postcompetition tests with little fear of detection. Drug abuse among athletes was allowed to blossom.

I want to emphasize that the unreliability of the testing prior to 1983 should not be attributed to human error in any way. Testing physicians wanted to do a good job. In essence, however, they were fighting the battle with an unloaded gun.

The inaccuracy of dope testing technology prior to 1983 resulted in both false positive results and a high number of false negatives. The false negative, where drugs were actually present but were not found in testing, was an extremely serious detriment to the testing process. When athletes knowingly used drugs, were tested, and were not found positive, it sent the message that their samples weren't really analyzed after all or that the tests were no good. Therefore, many athletes became adept at using their drugs and slipping through the cracks.

Even positive tests were met with intense scrutiny. An athlete who tested positive immediately appealed the decision, often using the unreliability of the testing process to get off the hook. When the laboratory director was asked on appeal to prove that the athlete was indeed using a banned substance ''beyond reasonable doubt,'' he or she could not, simply because of the inherent unreliability of the technology used in the testing process.

In addition, because the tests were unreliable, certain substances confused the analytical process and gave rise to certain ridiculous myths. For example, it was said that if someone ingested a dinner roll covered with poppy seeds, it could cause a positive test for heroin. Also, it was claimed that a commonly prescribed drug such as ibuprofen could be misinterpreted as a stimulant. This unreliability was one very effective argument against the infallibility of drug testing.

Perhaps the biggest opportunity to challenge the testing system at that time was the collection process itself: The handling or chain of custody of the after-competition urine samples could not be verifiably trusted to be tamperproof. Coding systems for specimen bottles were not well organized or kept confidential. The methods of pouring the urine into the specimen bottles were sloppy—another reason challenges based on possible contamination were upheld. Sealing methods had to be perfected: The wax used to seal the collection vials often cracked after refrigeration, leaving question as to whether the sample had been opened before analysis. Often, shy testing officials would not actually witness the athlete urinate; this allowed for all sorts of ways to beat the system.

When I first became involved in the testing program, I was witness to some almost unbelievable attempts by athletes to beat the system. Some tried catheterization to insert bogus urine into the bladder. Female athletes tried to beat the tests by inserting condoms filled with ''clean'' urine into their vaginas, then poking the condoms with pins to release the urine into the collection vials. Male athletes tried placing plastic bags filled with clean urine under their armpits or in the crack between their legs, with a tube leading to their penises. Some tried drinking copious amounts of water or taking a diuretic to dilute their own urine. One of the females' favorite tricks was scooping up toilet bowl water, proving that the hand could be quicker than the eye. Drug testers have since begun to dye toilet water blue in case a ''magician'' shows up for a drug test.

These are only a few of the bizarre methods once used by athletes to beat the testing, and some of these tricks are still being used today. When collection standards aren't scrupulously followed, violators manage to beat the system. This is especially true when the act of urinating is not witnessed, a major problem in all testing, including preemployment and workplace testing.

Therefore, one of my first duties after I took over the drug testing program for the USOC was to streamline this process to eliminate the loopholes inherent in the old system. Today all athletes are witnessed giving their sample, thereby eliminating the possibility of dilution or initial tampering by the athlete. Athletes are informed of their legal rights regarding the testing process, protocol, appeals, and so on from the time they first give a urine sample. The sealing and coding systems have also been improved to negate all questions concerning the validity of the collection process and the chain of custody. These changes have effectively enhanced the legal strength of the testing programs today.

Because the testing in years past did not include these details, it couldn't stand in the theater of amateur sport federation appeals nor, indeed, in any court of law. Without a strong legal foundation, built of reliable accuracy, these drug testing procedures were extremely weakened as a deterrent to drug use among athletes.

The athletes knew better than anyone that the drug testing posed little threat to them. They scoffed at testing notices and went right on with their routine drug use with little fear of detection.

Even the testers were intimidated by the deficient technology. This gave rise to a less libelous approach to testing called sink testing, used to prevent false positive reporting and legal challenges. This now nonexistent method meant all samples were collected but either were not tested or were simply poured down the drain.

Although athletes were known to be using substances to enhance performance, they all consistently came up negative in after-competition tests. It didn't really seem to matter exactly why or how they used their drugs: They always seemed to pass the tests. Whether samples were analyzed or just poured down the sink didn't seem to matter, because all tests came up negative.

Now, this may seem to have been a dishonest practice on the part of the testers, but that wasn't necessarily the case. It is understandable why, when dealing with an empty deck, the testers opted to take the sink testing route. It was less complicated. It avoided a potentially messy, unwinnable appeal. Nobody was falsely accused, nor was anyone hurt, and no legal complications occurred. It was difficult for good people to strip a gold medal from an individual if the tests were less than perfect.

Notwithstanding the con job, sink testing was still a deterrent in itself. Not knowing whether or not their specimens would be tested served as a threat to some naive athletes. The testing practice, though in many cases inefficient, at least raised in the minds of some athletes the potential of being caught. Thus, many athletes wouldn't chance it, and they avoided drug use altogether. So the testing wasn't completely ineffective, meaning there was still reason for the testing to exist.

I should also note that despite the shortcomings of the testing technology prior to 1983, some positive tests were obtained in international after-competition testing. I have already explained how American distance swimmer Rick DeMont lost his gold medal in the Munich Games of 1972 for testing positive for ephedrine, a stimulant drug found in many commonly used medications.

Nonetheless, cases like DeMont's were the exception, not the rule. Testing for stimulant drugs was fairly accurate, but the testing was not a real threat to athletes using other drugs. Particularly with anabolic-androgenic steroids, analysis had not been well researched or developed before that time. Furthermore, the technology available to drug testers was not reliable, sophisticated, or accurate enough to detect various AAS, testosterone, or its derivatives.

That all changed in 1983.

Before the 1983 Pan-American Games in Caracas, Venezuela, Professor Manfred Donike of Cologne, West Germany—using the biochemical research of such experts as Professor Raymond V. Brooks of London—put together a milestone program that dramatically changed the role drug testing played in the world of amateur sport. Professor Donike set the stage for the present, sophisticated, state-of-the-art drug testing in sport by implementing gas chromatography and mass spectrometry (GC/MS) in the analytical process.

The $30,000 gas chromatograph screens a small portion of the urine sample that an athlete provides. As a stream of helium gas sweeps the urine through a long tube, a detector registers a peak on a graph whenever it spots molecules that contain nitrogen or phosphorus, components of almost every banned drug. The time that the peak takes to appear reflects the time that the substance needs to pass through the tube, which in turn gives a strong hint as to the nature of the substance that produced the peak.

When technicians see a peak that seems to correspond to an illegal drug, they run another portion of the urine sample through a mass spectrometer, a $200,000 instrument that fragments molecules into easily recognized pieces. The instrument acts like an unerring fingerprint expert: If fragments in the urine sample fit the pattern of a banned drug programmed into the machine, the test is positive.

Maybe it is easier to understand this technology with the following analogy. Suppose someone is sorting through a pile in the junkyard, looking for a part of a vehicle. She initially comes across a glob of metal and rubber that she thinks may be a vehicle, so she picks it up and breaks it apart. Then she sees spread on the ground a collection of vehicle parts. By looking at these different parts, she sees a red truck body, a hook and

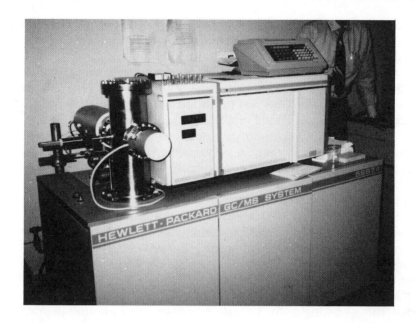

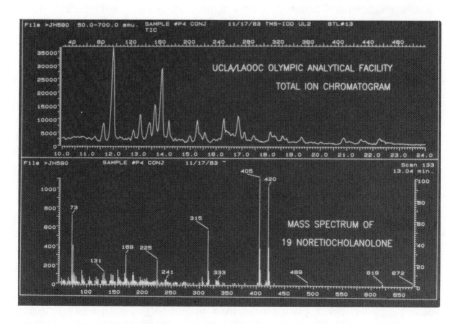

A new era of drug testing began in 1983 with the implementation of gas chromatography and mass spectrometry (GC/MS). Pictured here are a) a GC/MS testing system, and b) a readout analyzing a urine sample.

ladder, a water pump, and a hose. Without having to put the parts together, she has now discovered that the glob of metal and rubber, minus all the rust and debris, could be a fire engine.

At this point, the investigator might want to closely analyze these parts individually to determine whether they were originally part of one truck. She finds that the engine was produced in Detroit in 1956 and that the pump motor was produced in 1956. By further analysis of all the parts, she can then confirm without any doubt that this onetime glob was, at an earlier point, one fire engine. Not only has this person found a vehicle, but she knows exactly what type of vehicle it is.

Drug testing officials are able to learn the same type of information about chemical agents when using gas chromatography/mass spectrometry. Because this technology is so exquisitely accurate and is the standard in the world for use in forensic medicine and toxicology, positive drug tests can be made known publicly. The results of such a detailed process of drug testing are virtually indisputable. The results withstand scrutiny by all the world's courts.

Going into the 1983 Pan-Am Games, some athletes were doing their usual thing—taking anabolic-androgenic steroids and other performance enhancing drugs to prepare for competition—with little fear of being caught. Beating the tests and getting by with using drugs was a well-established science known by many athletes, coaches, and trainers. It was also widely discussed by the USOC Sports Medicine Council, but no substantial organized attempt was made by sport governing bodies to curtail the problem.

This is not by any means to say that the USOC medical staff condoned drug use among athletes. In fact, Dr. Daniel Hanley, of New Brunswick, Maine—then a member of the International Olympic Medical Commission and the first Olympic team physician—had been working on the problem of substance abuse among athletes for most of his professional career. Dr. Irving Dardik, then chairman of the USOC Sports Medicine Council, was also quite aware of the existence of drug problems among athletes and had spoken publicly condemning drug use and encouraging establishment of better detection methods. Dr. Roy Bergman, a general surgeon and a USOC Sports Medicine Council member from Michigan, was the appointed head physician for the Pan-American Games; he, too, had a good working knowledge of the drug problem.

Yet, as I have mentioned, considering the lack of effectiveness of drug testing and its known limitations, even the USOC Sports Medicine Council paid little heed to the threat of international testing before 1983. In some respects, the Council was torn over the issue of testing: Some wanted to do more to solve the problem, yet all realized our athletes needed these drugs in order to keep up with foreign competition.

The American medical staff went to Caracas before the Pan-Am Games to tackle an enormous list of potential problems before the competition got under way. Advance parties had reported that sanitary and domestic conditions were very poor in Caracas. There was great concern over whether or not foodstuffs and living conditions would cause various gastrointestinal ailments, if not upper respiratory illnesses, among the athletes. The medical staff was on a fact-finding mission to help counter these potential problems.

This gave Dr. Hanley the opportunity to investigate the drug testing lab. What he found, almost unexpectedly, was the most sophisticated laboratory capable of accurate anabolic-androgenic steroid testing in sport at that time. In Dr. Hanley's opinion, the laboratory was the hottest available in the world, capable of detecting all the banned substances, including caffeine and testosterone, which in years before had been very difficult for any laboratory to detect. It was also obvious to Dr. Hanley that there would be a tremendous number of athletes who would be surprised, caught off guard, and detected by this new sophisticated laboratory. He then proceeded to alert the medical staff that the testing would indeed be accurate and that the time for effective doping control had arrived.

Yet, some were skeptical, so Dr. Hanley invited medical staff member Dr. James Betts, a pediatric surgeon from San Francisco, to tour the facility. Dr. Betts agreed that rigid standards had been set up and the new technology applied by Professor Donike was, in fact, like nothing that had been seen before. Other members of the medical staff, including Dr. Bergman and Dr. Robert Leach, also toured the facility and were convinced from what they saw that the drug testing facility in Caracas was among the most sophisticated in the world. The medical staff quickly realized the possible effects this could have on unsuspecting athletes.

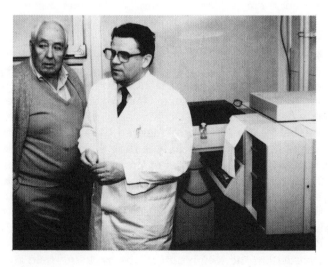

Dr. Hanley (left) inspecting an IOC drug testing lab.

The antidrug attitude leading up to those days was ridiculous. At that time, the USOC relied on the athletes' affidavits that they were drug free. With this as the primary weapon against drug use, there wasn't a very impressive deterrence program, but that was all the USOC had to go on.

"Are you on drugs?"

"Nope."

"You swear?"

"Yep."

"Will you put it in writing?"

"Sure."

"Fine."

That's basically all it was.

Of course, all the American athletes who had made the Pan-Am team denied banned drug use. This was the way things went in those days. Sport administrators were well aware of the tremendous use of anabolic-androgenic steroids and other drugs in sport, but nothing was being done to stop it.

The Pan-American medical staff, sensing the possibility of a major exposé, felt obliged to gather athletes, coaches, and managers to inform them that the new lab was fully capable of detecting all banned substances, including anabolic-androgenic steroids and testosterone.

Now, I must interject here that in most cases, medical staff recommendations would be followed, but unfortunately not when it came to drug use and testing. If the doctors said, "Don't drink the water," the athletes said, "OK." If the doctors said, "Don't use the drugs," well, that was a different story.

I have already described how, when anabolic-androgenic steroids were first introduced, there were few scientific studies that described why and how AAS worked. The medical profession in general explained naively that the effects of these drugs were probably more psychological than physiological. Thus, even in the early 1980s, many athletes thought physicians didn't know what they were talking about. The athletes perceived these warnings to be mere scare tactics. Some physicians, and most coaches and trainers, still felt anabolic-androgenic steroid use posed no health risk whatsoever.

Therefore, before the 1983 Pan-American Games, the athletes did not fully trust anything physicians said regarding anabolic-androgenic steroid use, and many were very skeptical of this recent revelation of new and highly accurate testing resources they were to encounter in Caracas. When Dr. Bergman and Dr. Leach presented the facts—that this situation posed a potential problem to the American delegation—some athletes countered by accusing the doctors of not knowing what they were talking about. They said, "You were wrong before, so why should we believe you now?" In particular, the weight lifters, the track-and-field athletes, and the physicians who were associated with these teams resisted the information that athletes might be at risk.

It was common knowledge at the time that practically 100 percent of the weight lifters had been involved with anabolic-androgenic steroids. Some had stopped their anabolic-androgenic steroid use only days or weeks before the Games. So, it appeared that because of the new, accurate testing facility being prepared in Caracas, the United States delegation was headed for an imminent public relations disaster.

Unable to make an impact with their warnings to these athletes, the medical staff took the responsibility to advise Colonel F. Don Miller, then the executive director of the USOC, of the potential problem. Once Colonel Miller was brought into this situation, the decision was made among all concerned parties that at least a screening urine test should be done before the Games actually got under way. The weight lifters were allowed to submit to these tests on a voluntary, anonymous basis, and they were to determine their own code numbers. The object was to allow the athletes an opportunity to make up their own minds as to whether they wished to chance disqualification.

After the samples were collected, they were sent to the same laboratory to be used in Caracas. But the agreement was to screen only, and only for anabolic-androgenic steroids and testosterone. The results were then reported to the athletes, and their rights were explained to them.

The U.S. delegation had reached Caracas, but many athletes left the Games and returned to the United States upon getting their results. As reported by UPI, they included Mark Patrick, 400-meter hurdles; Randy Williams, long jump; Brady Crain, sprinter; Paul Bishop and Greg McSeveny, discus; Dave McKenzie and John McArdle, hammer throw; Duncan Atwood, javelin; Mike Marlow, triple jump; and Gary Bastien, decathlon. Many gave reasons other than fears of drug testing to explain their absence.

Why did other athletes, though, knowing they were in danger of being detected for drug use by the testing, still choose to compete? One explanation given to me was that certain agreements had been made with the international federations to test only those athletes who won medals.

It appears now that such a secret agreement may have been reached for the weight lifting competition. In the pre-Games screening, nine of the weight lifters had tested positive for anabolic-androgenic steroids or testosterone, one tested negative, and one sample was too dilute to detect anything. Yet, none of the weight lifters left Caracas when given these results. Many of the weight lifters saved face simply by competing but not lifting enough to total, therefore not winning medals and not being officially tested in Caracas.

Jeff Michels, the American heavyweight weight lifter, however, went on to win three gold medals. He and a female judo competitor were the only two American athletes caught by the drug testing. He was disqualified and stripped of his medals.

The August 25, 1983, edition of *The Australian* reported that the Pan-American Games saw, in the words of former USOC President William Simon, "the largest expulsion of athletes in the history of international competition for drug abuse." A total of 21 medals were stripped from athletes, 11 of them gold. In addition to Michels, medals were stripped from weight lifters Alberto Blanco of Cuba, Michel Viau of Canada, Guy Greavette of Canada, Jacques Oliger of Chile, Enrique Montiel of Nicaragua, and Jose Adarmez Paez of Venezuela. Juan Nunez, a 100-meter sprinter from the Dominican Republic, was also stripped of his silver medal.

The same article in *The Australian* reported, "Although there was no hard evidence that the American track and field athletes left because they feared the new sophisticated drug laboratory might reveal that they were using illicit drugs, this fact was virtually confirmed by javelin thrower Curtis Ransford, the lone member of the eight-man Australian team who was still entered in the competition. Ransford later said, 'I knew there was going to come a day when no one could hide from the testing. Now they have the equipment, and this was the competition they decided to try it out on. It was the start of the new testing procedure.'"

Ransford, however, was not entirely correct in his statement that this was a first. Professor Donike had used the gas chromatography/mass spectrometry technology a month before the Pan-Am Games at the track-and-field World Championships in Helsinki. This fact is very interesting because the International Amateur Athletic Federation (IAAF) has always contended that there were no positives in Helsinki. If that was true, why then did so many athletes, most of whom competed a month before in Helsinki, leave the Pan-Am Games? What were the results in Helsinki?

I now know there were indeed positives in Helsinki that the IAAF covered up. Professor Donike admitted recently before the Dubin Inquiry (the Canadian government investigation into drug use after the Ben Johnson affair erupted in Seoul) that there were indeed positives. This verified what everyone but IAAF officials believed at the time. And this could quite possibly be the deciding reason for the mass exodus of U.S. track athletes from Caracas. Perhaps they were found positive in Helsinki but not disciplined. When they were told that they would not be treated with the same clemency in Caracas, however, they wisely chose to leave the competition.

Most of us interested in stopping drug use in sport were convinced that something very fishy happened in Helsinki. The IAAF didn't improve its image in regards to repressing drug test results by the way testing was handled at the 1987 track-and-field World Championships in Rome. I'll get back to this later.

Why Jeff Michels competed, and medaled, in Caracas has always been the subject of many questions. Through subsequent discussions with several members of the 1983 Pan-Am medical staff, I learned that Michels was the lone weight lifter whose sample had turned up negative in the initial, precompetition screening. After his event, though, his samples were positive.

Was this the result of a false negative in the precompetition screening? No one can be sure, but I would speculate that this situation was due to the body's strange, sometimes unpredictable excretion of anabolic-androgenic steroids. The level of excretion of AAS follows a sawtooth downward curve over time, meaning some days the drug is visible, and on others it may not be (see Figure 3).

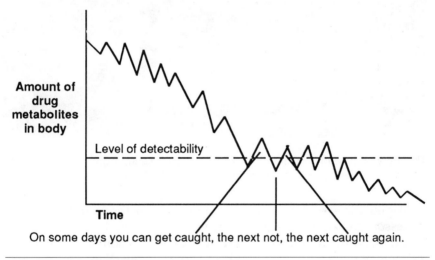

On some days you can get caught, the next not, the next caught again.

**Figure 3.**   Sawtooth curve.

It is possible that Michels could have cleared the first screening on a down day, at the bottom of an individual tooth on the curve. On the day he competed, his metabolites then may have been at the top level of a tooth. This serves as an example of the fickle nature of an individual's metabolism of drugs and as a caveat to the gurus, who also know that no two persons react with the same metabolic excretion rate of drugs. This is a fact that has surprised many drug users who have tested positive in competition.

Considering the knowledge the medical staff had in hand leading up to the 1983 Pan-American Games and the fact that anabolic-androgenic steroid use was rampant, the decision made by F. Don Miller, Dr. Bergman, and Dr. Leach to advise the team of the potential pitfalls that awaited them in Caracas was correct at the time. Today, though, such a decision would be considered highly unethical under the circumstances, considered in some respects aiding and abetting the cheaters.

All this was the scene as I joined the USOC as the chief medical officer. A new era of drug testing had begun, and the United States Olympic Committee was quite embarrassed.

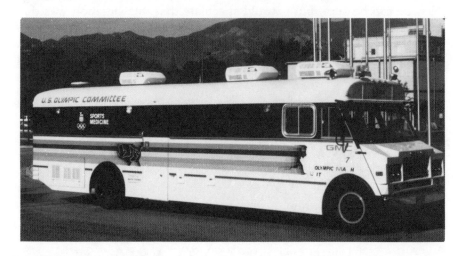

This mobile drug unit, acquired in 1985, was one result of the USOC efforts to expand its drug control efforts following the 1983 Pan American Games.

Despite the accuracy of the revolutionary methods introduced by Professor Donike in Caracas, a new era of avoiding detection had also begun. As with most actions, there had been a reaction: Out of this new technology evolved new methods of avoiding detection.

Despite the fact that the gas chromatography/mass spectrometry technology can identify banned substances in the urine in minute quantities (one part per billion) by molecular weight, human ingenuity is still able to beat most tests. One obvious method is for athletes to learn the excretion time for various substances. The athletes stop using these drugs in time to let their bodies clear the substances from their systems, but not too soon to lose their positive effects. Another method is to use growth hormone and other drugs that are invisible to present urine testing technology. The study of these methods has become the first task of doping gurus, who advise the athletes on how to use doping to their benefit.

Unfortunately, after the Pan-Am Games in Caracas, the intention and cautious nature of USOC policymakers in their initial application of drug testing played right into the hands of the gurus. In wishing to be fair and to educate athletes in the testing procedure, the initial program allowed for informal testing of athletes, with no sanctions leveled for positives. Thus, the national teams used frequent USOC testing. Because the purpose wasn't to expose users but to screen the athletes before given competitions, those found positive could discreetly withdraw, feigning injury or illness. This avoided an on-site exposé, such as the one in Caracas. Ultimately, this USOC drug testing program became just another tool the gurus and athletes could use to help them cheat.

I have always approached drug testing as a means to make the playing field level. Drug testing should be a tool to provide an environment for fair play. To do that, I try to detect any cheating at any time in any place. Yet, there are those who think testing should be less aggressive. So long as everyone appears clean at any given event, nobody gets embarrassed and nobody gets hurt.

This latter attitude was prevalent among many U.S. sport officials prior to the 1984 Olympic Games in Los Angeles. It was also the reason the Canadians criticized the USOC program. The Canadians alleged that our program was simply a screening program to clean up our athletes before they competed, much like the programs the Soviets and East Germans are known to have used to prepare their athletes for international competitions.

For example, in 1988 the Soviets were accused of having a ship floating off the shore of Korea to do the final screening of their athletes. *Zmena,* an official publication of the Communist Party of the Soviet Union, did admit in March 1989 that the Soviets indeed had a $2.5-million testing facility floating 60 kilometers from Seoul on board the ship *Michail Shalokhov* during the 1988 Olympic Summer Games. Evidently, some athletes were barred from participating in the Olympics because they would have failed after-competition tests. Those who tested positive were kept from moving into the Olympic Village and competing for the Soviet Union; injury or illness were the reasons given for the athletes' withdrawals.

Some of my athlete sources told me that in Calgary, Soviet skier Allai Levandi withdrew from the 1988 Olympic Winter Games after his trainers told him, "You've suddenly gotten a terrible stomachache—you understand?" I suspect the understanding was that his screening tests had come back positive.

The informal tests the USOC used for educational purposes were done away with in early 1984. The USOC officially stopped this program as soon as it discovered that athletes were using these tests to gauge when to stop taking banned substances in time to clear their systems before testing. All tests at the American Olympic Trials in 1984 were supposedly considered formal, meaning anyone who tested positive for banned substances would be disqualified and punished accordingly. If true, the criticisms of the Canadians and other delegations regarding the USOC testing procedures would have been unfounded.

Although I was not then privy to the results, at that time I thought most athletes who tested positive for banned substances at the 1984 Olympic Trials were disqualified. I have since heard differently. Not *all* who were tested and came up positive were disqualified. This question resurfaced in 1989 when sprinter Diane Williams, remarking about the situation in the world of track and field leading up to the '84 Games, suggested that many anabolic-androgenic steroid users from the United States competed in the 1984 Olympics. I've learned from other athletes that federation officials may have intentionally suppressed test results. Today we are uncovering a history of corruption, cheating, scandal, and politics that may have silently damaged many sports beyond our worst fears.

In a sense, we've only begun to chip away at the tip of the iceberg.

# 6

# Idle Threat

## Why Drug Testing Just Isn't Working

One of the sad lessons sports-world doping control officials are learning is just how ineffective drug testing policies in sport *still* are. Obviously, despite technological advances, we've left gaping holes in the process that violators continue to slip through.

Perhaps the weakest link in this chain are the lengthy warnings athletes are given before some types of drug tests are actually administered. Put it this way. Someone is told on December 11 that on January 11 a policeman will be waiting at the end of his driveway to check his driver's license. If his license has expired, he will probably be sure to have it renewed by January 11. Only a fool would not have things in order when he runs into the policeman.

In a sense, drug testing practices allow the athlete the same generous warnings. Today nearly all athletes know when they will be tested, and they know how to clear drugs from their bodies in order to pass the tests. Consequently, many testing programs seem to catch only the very foolish or unlucky athletes.

I have often been criticized for my own vocal criticism of advance-notice drug testing programs, the type of programs still used by many amateur and professional sport organizations in the United States. The NCAA drug testing program, most professional sports' testing programs, and many USOC-backed testing programs require lengthy advance warning. That's why they don't work and are a waste of money.

Admittedly, I had much to do with establishing announced testing in sport. But as I learned more about drug testing and the methods athletes use to beat these tests during my time as director of Sports Medicine and Science at the USOC, I realized how ineffective advance-notice testing is when it is the only tool used to fight the problem of anabolic-androgenic steroids. I learned that although advance-warning testing is an effective way to detect and thus deter the use of performance enhancing stimulants such as amphetamine and cocaine, if it is the only method used to control doping in sport, it will not in a million years solve the anabolic-androgenic steroid problem we see among American athletes.

The reason this type of testing is effective on one front and not the other needs to be clarified. Sport officials fail to understand the distinction between effective testing for stimulants and effective testing for anabolic-androgenic steroids. Quick-acting, rapidly excreted performance enhancing stimulants such as amphetamine and cocaine are able to pass through the body system in a relatively short period of time. An athlete takes these drugs to give himself or herself quick energy and endurance and to allay fatigue. Therefore, these substances are taken only minutes to hours before competition time.

If an athlete takes amphetamine a week before his race, for example, that drug will have no positive effect whatsoever on the date of competition. For amphetamine to be an effective performance enhancing drug, an athlete would have to take this stimulant just prior to his event, and the benefits of amphetamine would be experienced only during his event.

Yet, in after-competition testing, an athlete is asked to produce a urine sample for laboratory analysis immediately after having competed. In the example, drug testers would be able to detect the amphetamine in the athlete's after-competition urine sample because, though rapid in action, amphetamine simply cannot clear the body quickly enough to escape detection in the test. The athlete is unable to benefit from the drug unless he takes it within the time period when testing will detect use.

As I have mentioned, all substances clear the body in a certain amount of time. We gauge the amount of time needed to pass a substance from the body by its half-life. Each chemical substance has its own unique half-life: In testing, it is that period of time it takes the body to metabolize and excrete 50 percent of the given substance.

For example, alcohol has a half-life of approximately 20 to 30 minutes. If someone drinks one beer, in 20 to 30 minutes 50 percent of the alcohol in the beer will have been passed through the body. In another 20 to 30 minutes, 50 percent of what is left (meaning 25 percent of the original alcohol level) will have cleared the system. In general, it takes about five or six of these half-lives for a given chemical substance or drug to pass through the system virtually completely. Any amount left will be too small to be detected by laboratory analysis.

In the case of amphetamine, the elimination time is much longer, and its metabolites can be found up to 48 hours after use.

Anabolic-androgenic steroids have even longer half-lives than stimulants, meaning it takes longer for the body to eliminate them. The half-lives of these drugs can be days or weeks, not hours or minutes. To complicate this further, a lot of what determines the various half-lives of anabolic-androgenic steroids depends on whether the drugs are water soluble or given in an oil-based form. Oil-based AAS can sometimes take months to completely clear the athlete's system. However, the water soluble anabolic-androgenic steroids taken in tablet form usually clear in a matter of weeks. Both forms of AAS are taken during the athlete's training period to build muscle. The effects of anabolic-androgenic steroids are not achieved immediately, unlike stimulant effects. Therefore, many athletes "stack" both oil-based and water-soluble anabolic-androgenic steroids in huge doses to maximize muscle gains.

Let's look at what happens when an athlete uses the anabolic-androgenic steroid Deca-Durabolin. Deca-Durabolin, also known by its generic name, nandrolone, or in gym parlance simply as Deca is one of the most popular AAS because of its long, smooth action associated with great gains. Deca, however, is an oil-based injectable anabolic-androgenic steroid. It has a long elimination time. In my experience, I have seen athletes test positive for nandrolone months after a single dose. In fact, as I said earlier, I have witnessed several cases where nandrolone is still detectable 12 to 18 months after use.

Now, an athlete must stop taking a given drug so that the AAS will clear his body in time to pass the postcompetition drug test but not so soon that the positive effects will wear off. The positive effects of anabolic-androgenic steroids aren't permanent, decreasing steadily after use is discontinued, even when the necessary strength training is continued. For AAS to be effective, the athlete has to know how to take them; otherwise, the competitive edge won't last long enough to make a difference. This, one can see, is where the art of using anabolic-androgenic steroids can be a tricky business.

So, announcing to the athlete when he or she will be tested makes it a lot simpler to figure out what types of anabolic-androgenic steroids to use and when to stop using them in order to test negative. By giving lengthy advance notice of testing to competitors, all we do is help the drug users gauge exactly when to discontinue steroid use before a given competition. After-competition drug testing is still necessary if stimulant use is to be prevented. With regard to anabolic-androgenic steroid use, however, only a combination of continuous, frequent event testing and testing during training periods before key events will deter use.

The science of avoiding drug detection is probably as sophisticated today as the science of drug testing itself. From what athletes tell me, I know that the drug users continue to be about a lap ahead of the testing initiative in almost all circumstances. The resources and effort poured into the study of avoiding detection can, at times, be almost unbelievable. Anabolic-androgenic steroid users actually have clandestine laboratories at their disposal, which they can use for screening, determining the amount of substance to use, and planning when to get off these substances to clear a drug test. They have physicians, exercise physiologists, pharmacologists, and very experienced drug users who are willing to serve as their steroid gurus and teach them the various tricks to avoid detection. These gurus prey on athletes at various gyms and fitness centers throughout the country, in virtually every community, big and small.

Generally, competitions at the elite level of amateur sport always invite athletes to participate in their events. That means the athletes receive written notices of sorts months in advance of the competition dates. Those letters usually contain some notification of testing policies for that event, and the athletes invited are therefore given every opportunity to clear their systems of banned substances. Any potential effectiveness of an advance-warning drug testing policy is thereby nullified.

I have seen many situations where, if for some reason caught off guard without previous knowledge of testing policies, athletes simply withdraw from their events rather than fail the drug test. There have been numerous, documented cases, particularly in track and field and weight lifting, where many athletes have registered to compete in events months before they began, yet, once they reported and found out that there would be drug testing, they suddenly left the competitions in swarms. The exodus from the 1983 Pan-American Games was an excellent example of this, although in this case the athletes knew they would be tested: They just didn't realize how good the testing would be.

There have been more recent examples. The Gatorade Track and Field Classic, held in Knoxville, Tennessee, in May 1988, happened to be scheduled months before the Olympic Games. However, this event came during the anabolic-androgenic steroid cycling phase when athletes were gearing up for the U.S. Olympic Trials in Indianapolis. Many of the athletes were in the final stages of their training cycles.

When the athletes were informed of the drug testing that would take place in Knoxville, many withdrew from the competition. Of eight discus throwers registered for the meet, one showed up. Of nine athletes entered in the shot put event, only four showed up. A premiere American triple jumper decided at the last minute not to compete.

In my opinion, the only explanation for this incredibly high dropout rate is that these athletes were juicing (taking anabolic-androgenic steroids) at the time and they wanted neither to fail a drug test nor to cease the use of their AAS before the Trials.

A second example is the 1988 Pepsi Classic, an international track-and-field meet scheduled to take place weeks before the Olympic Trials. Because testing was to be done at the Pepsi Classic, many athletes did not accept their invitations to compete. The shot put and discus events at the Pepsi Classic had to be cancelled.

This situation, I believe, is one of the reasons several amateur sport federations, particularly those governing track and field, judo, and weight lifting, have been reluctant in the past to fully endorse aggressive drug testing programs. These federations depend on international competitions as a major part of their fund-raising efforts. They don't like the notion of mandatory drug testing at every international competition held in this country because testing negatively affects the athlete attendance at a meet. And when the big guns don't show up for an event, the fans don't show up either.

Most athletes with a decent understanding of the elimination time of the substance they're using, a drug testing notice, and a calendar will pass almost any advance warning drug test around. If all else fails, they are still able to walk away from the event rather than take the test.

Considering all this, however, I am often asked, "Why, then, would an athlete get caught for anabolic-androgenic steroid use if drug testing is announced in a way that allows the athlete time to cease drug use long enough in advance of the competition to clear the screening? How can you claim advance-notice testing is ineffective in stopping AAS use if we can still detect some users? How, for example, do you explain a world-class athlete like Ben Johnson testing positive for AAS in the 1988 Olympic Summer Games?"

I can postulate several fairly simple answers to these questions. We're dealing with a huge black market when we talk about anabolic-androgenic steroids. And the AAS gurus advising athletes on the use of these drugs, though they may know some tricks of the trade, aren't always the smartest physiologists in the world.

The human body is difficult to predict. It is sometimes very tricky to gauge the rate of hydration, the rate of excretion, and the metabolic rate of each individual (see the related discussion on Jeff Michels in chapter 5). There are many factors that can slow the excretion of anabolic-androgenic steroids from this highly complex machine. Individual metabolism, amount of substance used, frequency of use, length of time used, and the normal biodegradation process in any given individual will vary.

Many of the anabolic-androgenic steroids used today are oil-based and are stored in the body's fat deposits for an unknown period of time. In the precompetition training phase, a user may work hard enough to burn off some of this fat and metabolize stored AAS in the process. The metabolites then show up in the urine, though at times before this the urine may have been clear. It is possible, therefore, for an athlete to think that he or she is clean by having allowed a normally sufficient period of time for the drug to clear, only to find out that some time before the competition the intense training had mobilized more fat stores. The metabolites of these drugs will then pass through the urine in a way that allows detection.

Every athlete who uses anabolic-androgenic steroids is exposed to that risk. Usually, though—indeed, in most cases—the athlete is able to hit the mark with fair accuracy.

Another possible explanation is best described by using the analogy of an embezzler who is caught stealing from the bank. The embezzler rarely gets caught so long as he doesn't vary from his program of stealing. But the minute he starts taking just 10 dollars more, the red light goes on, signalling that something is wrong. The embezzler often will not get caught for the initial crime; rather, he'll be discovered after he's gotten a bit too greedy and is no longer consistent with his scheme.

The same can be said of some athletes who test positive for anabolic-androgenic steroid use. Athletes usually follow a routine anabolic-androgenic steroid program to a T. Say, for example, an athlete knows her body can clear the steroid she is taking within 21 days after she stops using it. When that 21-day clearing period finally begins, the athlete sometimes gets nervous and says to herself, ''Have I done enough? Will the effects last? Maybe if I can shrink the limit to 20 days, maybe if I can hang in there for just 24 hours longer, I'll have that little extra edge over my competition.'' And so, the athlete's insecurity sometimes deceives her into blowing her cover, much like the greed of the embezzler.

I would speculate that this is probably what happened to Ben Johnson. I suspect that Johnson just got greedy and thought he could take an extra dose of his anabolic-androgenic steroid (stanozolol) and get away with it. Before Seoul, Johnson knew that he and American Carl Lewis would probably compete in the fastest 100-meter dash in history. He also knew that winning that race would mean millions of dollars, fame, and an entirely better way of life. One can only imagine the thoughts in Ben Johnson's mind in the days leading up to that race. This was Johnson's once-in-a-lifetime shot, and the importance of that competition was just too much for him not to take the gamble. Besides, in over 8 years of anabolic-androgenic steroid use, he had never been caught before.

Another reason an athlete might get caught using anabolic-androgenic steroids is from just not being smart enough to plan for the testing properly. Either the athlete or the guru didn't know enough about taking the drug, and they got caught out of plain ignorance.

Perhaps an athlete may just be too physically or psychologically addicted to the drug to stop.

One final reason is now that these athletes are using so many black market and European anabolic-androgenic steroids, they just can't be sure of exactly what they're getting anymore. In the old days, when the athletes were using anabolic-androgenic steroids produced primarily by large, reputable American pharmaceutical houses, they could be certain of the dose. Because of the strict quality control at the industrial level, they could also feel comfortable with the purity of what they were getting.

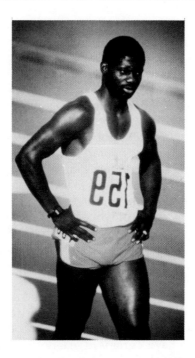

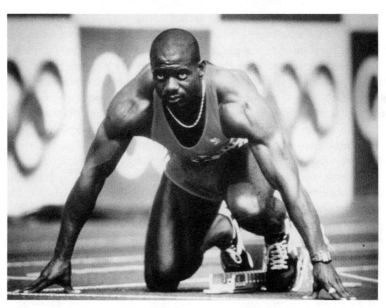

Ben Johnson's muscle development is apparent in these photos taken a) in 1982 at the Commonwealth Games, and b) in 1988 at the Olympics in Seoul.
*Note.* ©Allsport USA/Tony Duffy. 1982, 1988. Reprinted by permission.

Today, though, athletes might think that they are buying some exotic foreign anabolic-androgenic steroid, when in fact what they could be getting is a relatively common and inexpensive substitute, like ordinary testosterone. I have counseled athletes who have tested positive for a high testosterone ratio and have sworn to me that they had never used testosterone in their lives. After further investigation of their drug stories, I'd discover that instead of the anabolic-androgenic steroids they thought they had bought, they actually got only testosterone cypionate—at 10 times its normal price.

Because we're dealing with criminal sources for these drugs, it shouldn't come as a surprise to some that black market dealers sell cheap product for the highest possible price in order to secure a larger profit margin. To the black marketeer, that's only making a dirty business a bit dirtier.

For example, if someone wanted to buy a gram of cocaine on the street in Los Angeles, he'd be nuts if he thought he was going to buy 1 gram of pure cocaine. By the time the street dealer gets ahold of that gram, it will have passed through several people's hands. Each person who had handled the cocaine would have broken it up and added artificial powder (usually sugars, crushed breath mints, or local anesthetic powders) to increase the total mass and reduce the purity of the cocaine. That way, when they go to resell it, they have 2 grams to sell, not 1. That's how they double their money. By the time a buyer gets his gram, what he usually receives is one part cocaine, three parts tic-tac®.

Often anabolic-androgenic steroid black marketeers do a similar thing. Don't think for a minute the person selling these drugs cares one bit about athletes, their health, or how they perform on the playing field. The only thing that matters to these crooks is making money. Understandably, this poses a variety of risks to the athletes. If they can't be sure of the proper dosage and if they think they're taking something other than what they're really taking, they not only expose themselves to the risk of detection, but they may also seriously jeopardize their health, if not their lives.

One case where an unknown "miracle" drug proved to be lethal involved West German heptathlete Birgit Dressel. Aided by her religious use of anabolic steroids and other performance enhancing drugs, Dressel had risen in the heptathlon world rankings from 33rd to 6th—all within the period of just 1 year.

Dressel's drug program included various complex vitamins, pain medications, and anabolic-androgenic steroids. She had also received an anabolic drug named Megagrisevit in an anonymous post package. On April 7, 1987, driven by her quest to improve even more and desperate to find that one miracle drug that would put her on top, Dressel threw caution to the wind and added this Megagrisevit to her daily diet of medications.

On April 10, 1987, Dressel died from her body's violent rejection of the numerous drugs she took. Indeed, this Megagrisevit may have pushed her over the edge.

---

*Author's Note:*   This case has many other serious ramifications and will
be discussed again in chapter 8.

---

For the sake of the athletes, I sometimes wish the black market were
more reliable. Not because I want to see them cheat more effectively, but
because, as a physician, I am seriously concerned for the health of the
athletes who, like Dressel, are willing to gamble on unprescribed medications from the hands of unreliable black marketeers or steroid gurus.

To give you an idea of the number of substances athletes sometimes
take, I recorded one athlete's daily diet as follows: vitamin E, 1,600 mg;
B-complex capsules, four times per day; vitamin C, 2,000 mg; vitamin $B_6$,
150 mg; calcium tablets, four times daily; magnesium tablets, twice a day;
zinc tablets, three times a day; royal jelly capsules; garlic tablets; cayenne
tablets; eight aminos; Gamma-Oryzanol; Mega Vit Pack; supercharge
herbs; Dibencozide; glandular tissue complex; natural steroid complex;
Inosine; Orchic testicle extract; Pyridium; Ampicillin; and hair rejuvena-
tion formula with Biotin.

That was what the athlete admitted to taking. What banned drugs was
he also taking but unwilling to admit to? This was, by the way, a national
track star.

I hope we will ultimately be able to catch and severely punish those
operating the black market and avoid the problem altogether. To date,
though, very little has been done, and I can safely say that the black
market prospers.

Now, one might think that with all the potential ways an anabolic-
androgenic steroid user could be detected, drug testers should be catching more athletes than they are. That's just not the case. Most of the bright
athletes continue to get by the testing roadblocks. In my mind, the only
way to counter the health risks posed by anabolic-androgenic steroids
and to restore credibility to sport competitions is to enhance the effectiveness of drug testing programs nationwide.

The first step we're going to have to take in that direction is to stop
depending solely upon lengthy advance-warning drug testing practices.
We must maintain our effectiveness in fighting stimulant use with
postcompetition testing. But we also need to bolster the fight against
anabolic-androgenic steroids by developing additional alternatives to
advance-notice testing. This means we need to incorporate short-notice
testing and some forms of limited out-of-competition testing into the overall program.

Whether some of the officials who are in the position to make such
changes have the desire and fortitude to do so—well, only time will tell.
I know that in the past, many haven't.

# 7

# Testing Gone Afoul

## *Cover-ups, Lies, and Manipulation— All for the Sake of Gold*

Allowing national governing bodies (NGBs), international federations (IFs), and national Olympic committees (NOCs) such as the United States Olympic Committee to govern the testing process to ensure fair play in sport is terribly ineffective. In a sense, it is like having the fox guard the henhouse.

There is simply too much money involved in international sports today. One needs to understand that the officials in charge of operating sport at the amateur level need world-class performances to keep their businesses rolling forward. The sad truth is that people don't pay to watch losers, and corporations don't sponsor teams that can't bring home the gold. The athletes and officials realize this, so they're willing to do whatever it takes to win. And sometimes that means turning their backs on the drug problem.

When an international hero such as Ben Johnson is exposed for cheating, everyone—I mean *everyone*—feels repercussions from this blow. The sport federations lose money. They lose public interest and support. They are forced to face sharp, intense scrutiny from the media. Thus, many officials seem more willing to turn their backs on the problems, sweep them under the rug, and avoid an exposé rather than become a laughing-stock before the world.

Even a testing process that uses the most sophisticated scientific resources and is controlled by the most altruistic officers is therefore susceptible to manipulation. I have seen numerous cases where I suspect cover-ups to have taken place not only to protect the images of the violating athletes but also to protect the sport organizations in charge of maintaining a level of fair play.

Ultimately, turning the other cheek on these issues comes back to bite the parties involved on their rear ends. One needs to remember that by shielding the offenders, officials are really sending a negative message to the majority of athletes who have chosen to compete clean. Believe me when I say that the athletes know who is on "the juice" and who is not. When they see an individual who they know to be using drugs glide safely through a national or international competition without being exposed, how do you think the clean ones feel? How does the kid who got fourth at the Olympic Trials and missed making the team by .001 second feel when he knows the top three finishers were using drugs? How much does he value the support of his sport federation when he knows nothing is being done to stop the problem? What kind of a message does this send to the young athlete on the verge of making it big? It tells him to use drugs—to win, baby, win. Put up or shut up (or be lost in the gears of this machine forever).

I know from dealing directly with the athletes that most of them resent this situation. For this reason, I've decided to share some of my own questions concerning drug testing at major international sports competitions in recent years. Quite honestly, there are things that have happened over the past 8 years that I simply cannot explain. I think it is about time the world got some honest answers to these questions. The athletes and the sports fans around the globe deserve to know the truth. In my mind, if the individuals who govern sport today can't come up with the truth, we ought to find people for those positions who can.

Most of my examples for this discussion center on the world of track and field and the governing bodies controlling this sport on the national level (The Athletics Congress, or TAC) and the international level (International Amateur Athletic Federation, or IAAF). This is not because I have a personal vendetta against track and field. It is because, as you will soon see, this sport has what I believe to be the darkest history when it comes to drug abuse among athletes—and the unwillingness of officials to work effectively toward eliminating the problem.

Let's look first, for example, at an event I have already discussed in considerable detail, the 1983 Pan-American Games in Caracas, Venezuela. As I have said, the 1983 Pan-Am Games was one of the first international events where the sophisticated gas chromatography/mass spectrometry (GC/MS) testing analysis system was used to test athletes for doping violations. The GC/MS was extremely accurate, and the USOC doctors knew this was going to cause problems, particularly for the weight lifters. So the USOC decided to screen the weight lifting team for drug use and explain to those athletes who tested positive the potential courses of action they could take to avoid disqualification and sanctions in Caracas. Consequently, many of the weight lifters chose not to win medals at the Games.

There were also a number of American track-and-field athletes who, on the eve of competition, chose not to compete in the Pan-Am Games. The track-and-field athletes used flimsy excuses to explain their mass exodus from Caracas. Now, we know why the weight lifters chose to sidestep the testing in Caracas: They knew they would get caught by the drug testing lab at the Games site.

Evidently, the track and field team had the same insight. But how? The track team had not been screened by the USOC before the Pan-Am Games like the weight lifters. I also seriously doubt that word had spread through the athletes' village grapevine fast enough to have allowed the weight lifters to warn the track team, if they had even cared to. Somehow, certain athletes had been introduced to the GC/MS system. The athletes knew it worked. They also knew if GC/MS were to be used in Caracas, they would be caught. Because many of these athletes didn't want to take that chance, they simply left the Games.

So how did the track athletes get their information? Where did they learn that the tide had turned in the world of drug use and dope testing? Helsinki: the 1983 track-and-field World Championships. Just prior to the Pan-American Games, the gas chromatography/mass spectrometry system had been used at Helsinki. For some strange and mysterious reason, however, no athletes were found positive (or, as I should say, no positives were reported) at this meet. Somehow, the Helsinki testing alerted track and field to the effectiveness of the new testing.

---

*Author's Note:*   At the recent Dubin Inquiry in Canada, it was admitted that there were indeed positives in Helsinki.

---

This new testing—as a matter of fact, the very same equipment from Helsinki—was used a week later in Caracas. Considering that athletes virtually fled the 1983 Pan-Am Games for fear of this new dope testing equipment, how could so many positives turn up in Caracas when none had been turned up a week earlier in Helsinki? The known facts just don't add up! Why would the track athletes at the Pan-American Games fear a drug testing system that was unable to detect *any* violators at the World Championships?

The only explanation I can offer is the following. Some of the athletes in Caracas had also competed in Helsinki. There they tested positive, were told of the test results, and were let off the hook. The word was out, however, that anyone testing positive in Caracas would be reported and sanctioned. This happened probably because the Pan-American Organizing Committee was in charge of the testing the second time around, not the IAAF.

Did the IAAF choose to cover up the results in Helsinki? They must have. But reports of the effectiveness of the GC/MS system of testing were leaked to the athletes. I have heard that the track athletes were actually warned about the testing by a top USOC official before the events got under way. Realizing that the same equipment would be used in Caracas and that positives would *not* be treated with clemency there, many athletes decided to walk from the Pan-American Games.

A big problem here is that a number of world and national records were broken in Helsinki. How can we allow those records to stand if the competition was unfair because of the illegal use of banned substances? (Interestingly, the IAAF did strip Ben Johnson of the 100-meter world record he set at the 1987 World Championships in Rome after he admitted use of anabolic-androgenic steroids at the Dubin Inquiry in 1989. This seems ironic, considering the foul play that the IAAF allegedly allowed in Helsinki, and later in Rome.)

I am not the only person who is considerably suspicious about the drug testing game that was played in Helsinki. In fact, even International Olympic Committee Vice President Richard Pound of Canada, who many believe is the heir apparent to IOC President Juan Antonio Samaranch, said in regard to the testing in Helsinki, ''My feeling was that . . . there either were positives that were not acted upon by the IAAF or that there were directions not to test for certain compounds or substances.''[20]

So who was in the position to give such directions? Let's start from the top. The president of the IAAF is Primo Nebiolo of Italy. Nebiolo has been in the center of many disputes in the world of track and field. In fact, attempts were made to relieve Nebiolo of his duties as the president of the Italian Track and Field Association because of allegations that he had misappropriated funds for private contracts and because of his involvement with a scheme to add to the measurement of an Italian long jumper's leap at the 1987 track-and-field World Championships in Rome. Nebiolo is also one of the loudest opponents of standardized penalties for drug offenders. There is no doubt in my mind that, at least in 1983, Nebiolo would not have pressed for honest, accurate testing in Helsinki.

The next man to look at might be Dr. Arne Ljungquist of Sweden. As director of the IAAF Medical Commission, Ljungquist was actually in charge of the testing practices in Helsinki. Ljungquist, who has now come out publicly as a crusader in the fight against drugs, expressed his former attitude toward the testing process when he said, ''At the major meets, everybody knows samples will be taken and analyzed. So I don't expect to find positives.''[22] Suffice it to say that if someone told me Ljungquist were involved in planning a cover-up, I would not be at all surprised. I'll get back to him later.

The third player who could probably give us some answers to the World Championship mystery, but hasn't, is another vice president of the IAAF, Mr. Ollan Cassell (he was elected to this position in 1984 but was an IAAF council member during the Helsinki meet). An American, Cassell also happens to be the executive director of TAC. Actually, I have the utmost respect for Cassell's ability as a leader. He is private, intelligent, and dangerously effective. Perhaps his greatest credit is his heartfelt interest in looking after the rights of his athletes. However, I often got the sense when working with TAC that the better the athlete was, and the more press exposure the athlete could garner for TAC, the more this organization cared about his rights.

I am pretty sure that Cassell does not condone drug use; in fact, he has publicly stated many times that he believes drugs have no place in sport. But Cassell understands that he is living in the real world, meaning he knows drugs are, at this time, just part of the game. Now that the Ben Johnson situation has shocked the world about the present drug use among athletes, Cassell has become a ''born-again'' antidrug campaigner. To date, however, TAC's inability to formulate and enact an effective drug control program that its own athletes can trust and respect is, in my mind, a reflection of either insincerity or incompetence on behalf of TAC's leadership with regard to doping control.

That also says nothing about Cassell's past attitude and actions toward the drug problem. In 1985 I attended the organizing committee meeting of TAC's drug testing program, which was, oddly, called a ''protective testing program.'' Soon after the program was initiated, while supervising the agency that did some of TAC's collections, I began to seriously question whom this program was designed to protect. Working with TAC on the protective testing program, the USOC drug crews were often sent off to ''mom-and-pop'' track meets around the country. The meets chosen for testing were supposedly selected at random by a TAC computer. However, it seemed rather odd to me after a while that no matter where we went, we didn't seem to be drawing the ''big guns'' or the ''high-powered'' meets.

Who *were* we catching for drug use? A 58-year-old marathoner, who was on some needed medication. A 13-year-old junior runner. Those types of athletes. Certainly not elite track stars: We rarely saw them.

In fact, it soon became obvious to me that the big-name athletes knew damn well what events to stay out of and when. Somebody—I suspect some person inside TAC—had to have been tipping the athletes off. Who? We'll never know. Interestingly, in 1990 TAC announced its plan to conduct random short-notice out-of-competition testing. The athletes, however, tell me they are still not worried about beating the tests. Most of them say they can count on some source inside TAC to keep them informed of where, when, and how the tests will be conducted.

If, by chance, my drug testing crew were able to detect an elite athlete's drug use, there still seemed to be enough loopholes in the protective testing program to allow the athlete to get off the hook with little problem. That really irritated me. We could find an athlete positive for drug use and have him virtually nailed to the wall, only to watch him get off the hook on a technicality. Time and time again, Cassell and TAC president Frank Greenberg were the ones responsible for letting him go.

To Cassell's credit, he is a stickler for the legal rights of the individual. I have absolutely no argument against that: That's the American way. But if we allow an athlete who we *know* is guilty of a doping violation to go unpunished because a form wasn't filled out correctly or something, whose rights are we really protecting? No doubt, the violator is protected.

But what about the athlete who competes clean? What about Ms. Fourth Place? Shouldn't we place more emphasis on protecting and preserving a level of fairness for *all* competitors? Looking at past examples, it would appear as if TAC didn't think so. It's a money game, and they protected the ones who brought back the medals—the rest be damned. The legal rights of the cheaters have, in my mind, sometimes been used purely as smoke screens to hide behind.

For example, TAC got six premier American athletes, including shot-putter Augie Wolf and former world record pole-vaulter Billy Olson, off the hook in 1989 after both had tested positive for high testosterone levels. According to former USOC Substance Abuse Committee Chairman Edwin Moses, TAC torpedoed these athletes' drug hearings by providing the drug panels with deliberately insufficient information to counter biochemical defenses by the athletes. That way, the athletes were exonerated on legal grounds.[21]

In 1987 I had the opportunity to do the drug testing for the TAC National Outdoor Championships in San Jose, California. I was expecting to test 125 athletes at this event because I was told that 125 competitors would be tested. For reasons beyond my control, however, our urine sample collection lab was sent more athletes to be tested than the original number. I ultimately ran out of equipment before I could test 3 of the athletes who were designated to be tested.

Thus, I chose to have one of my colleagues, Harmon Brown, MD, the head of TAC's medical committee, conduct the tests on these athletes the following day because he had the necessary equipment right there in his office in San Jose. Dr. Brown had formerly been a USOC drug testing crew chief; he, like I, felt compelled to test the remaining 3 athletes to ensure that fair treatment had been given to all competitors. If we found drugs (particularly AAS) in the athletes' urine days *after* the meet, surely they would have been there during the meet as well.

Indeed, one of these athletes was found positive for the anabolic-androgenic steroid nandrolone. His name is John Powell, and he was the 1987 national champion in the discus. Dr. Brown had sent Powell's sample—an A sample and a B confirmation sample—to the drug testing lab at UCLA. Once the A sample was analyzed and recorded as positive, Powell, TAC officials, and the USOC were notified. Powell was then to appear at the B confirmation meeting, where the second sample would be analyzed. To make a long story short, the B sample also turned up positive, indicating that Powell was indeed guilty of a doping violation.

Cassell and other members of TAC, however, got Powell off the hook by appealing this decision on the basis that Dr. Brown made a technical error in coding the B sample, thus breaching USOC protocol. Dr. Brown, in labeling the specimen vials, marked Bottle A "XY05A" and Bottle B "XY5B." He accidentally omitted the "0" from the label on the second bottle. Dr. Brown also accidentally mailed the samples via the U.S. Postal Service without an attached Chain of Custody Form.

Due to these technicalities, Powell went scot-free, despite the fact that he had *personally signed* vial XY5B. In addition, the envopaks in which the samples were placed and mailed showed absolutely no signs of tampering. Powell had personally witnessed the sealing of these envopaks and had signed a form indicating that the process had been done correctly. When the envopak reached the UCLA lab for analysis, the seal had not been broken.

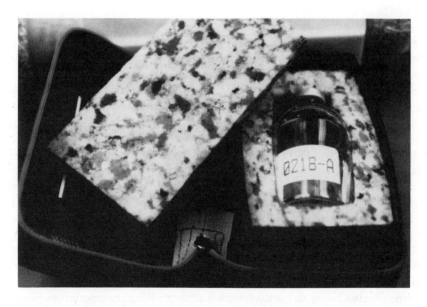

An envopak like the one Dr. Brown used to mail the specimen vials
from John Powell.

There is absolutely, positively no possible way that the urine in either Bottle A or Bottle B did not belong to Powell. He watched the urine come out of his body and go into the collection bottle. He watched the bottle be separated into two samples and sealed. He signed his name to indicate that the whole process had, in his own eyes, been handled correctly. Still TAC and USOC, in their infinite wisdom, saw reason to let Powell off the hook on the basis of one missing digit. Why? Because he was good, very good.

To make matters worse, during the testing process, Powell did not seem the least bit worried, concerned, upset, or remorseful. In fact, he went so far as to say, ''I don't care what you find. If you find something, so what?'' He must have known there were forces in his corner, forces that could protect him and set him free.

My question here, however, is why did TAC protect the athlete so well? Don't the interests of the many—the very concept of fairness in sport—outweigh the interests of one cocky drug user? How about the clean athletes who got beat by this guy? Don't you think TAC would feel compelled to help them? Evidently not, especially when there is a big international event on the horizon and TAC is thirsty for some medal production.

You see, all of this winds its way back to the international track scene, the IAAF, and the 1987 track-and-field World Championships in Rome. With his performance in San Jose, Powell earned a spot on the United States World Championship Team. Indeed, he traveled to Rome and won a medal in his event.

I know, from my experience in testing athletes, that Powell had enough nandrolone in his body at the time of our first test that he could not possibly have cleared the after-competition tests in Rome—that is, unless someone played around with the testing process.

IOC Medical Commission members Dr. Manfred Donike of West Germany and Dr. Arnold Beckett of Great Britain—who are, you will remember, the world authorities on gas chromatography/mass spectrometry drug testing—had volunteered and were scheduled to oversee the drug testing at the World Championships in Rome. Just weeks prior to the event, the IAAF Council decided to replace Donike and Beckett with two other doctors, Dr. Virginia Mikhaylova of Bulgaria and one Dr. Arne Ljungquist. Why the switch? I have yet to hear an explanation.

It was Dr. Ljungquist who officially reported no positives in Helsinki in 1983. In Rome in 1987 he reported one. Sandra Gasser of Switzerland, who won a bronze medal in the 1500 meters, was the only athlete the IAAF found guilty of a doping violation. She had used anabolic-androgenic steroids.

Was Gasser really the only positive athlete? What happened to Powell? There must have been a mistake somewhere, right? Many athletes have suggested to me that as many as 30 to 40 percent of the competitors in Rome were using drugs.

Did the IAAF brass, Nebiolo, Ljungquist, Cassell, and others reach an agreement not to test or not to report? Was there a cover-up? I think the evidence has to make you wonder. I, like many track-and-field athletes who competed in Rome, am still waiting for some answers. And I'm sure many sports fans around the world would also be interested in knowing just how legitimate the numerous national and world records set in Rome really are.

Another problem I have with TAC's protective testing program is the very length of the appeal process. Both TAC and the USOC allow athlete appeals to drag on for ridiculously long periods of time; this can be quite damaging. For example, the case of Powell was not fully resolved until November 1987, 5 months after the positive test in San Jose. In the meantime, Powell was allowed to go over and win a medal in Rome. That's wrong. If there's doubt—particularly, serious doubt, as there was in this case—you can't send that athlete to Rome in place of the kid who finished one place away from making the team but competed clean.

TAC and the USOC have another real weakness with regard to their approach to testing in the way they handle the issue of "innocent or inadvertent use." As I have explained before, an athlete found positive for ephedrine, or the derivatives of this drug commonly found in over-the-counter medications, may be excused on the premise that he or she accidentally used the drug. This is permitted on a one-time-only basis: The athlete can't make the same mistake twice (in international competition, the IOC grants no one-time pardons).

I have problems with this idea in that the athletes might be able to use this pardon to help them cheat with the full understanding that they would be let off the hook. Such could have been the case, I believe, with the 1988 U.S. Olympic Track and Field Trials in Indianapolis. There were eight analytically positive TAC athletes there. They were found positive for ma-huang, the herbal plant source for ephedrine, a banned central nervous system stimulant. The athletes involved were all excused for innocent use of a vitamin product that contained ma-huang. Had these athletes gone to Seoul (which they did) and tested positive for this substance (which they did not), it would have been a huge embarrassment to the United States—equal, I believe, in magnitude to the Ben Johnson situation.

The problem here, however, is that the athletes in question were not new to the testing process. They had been tested before, many times. They were well aware of the rules regarding ma-huang and other herbs. They also knew that the rules were such that if you "innocently" took these substances, you could be excused on a one-time-only basis. I was a member of the USOC appeal board that heard their appeal and didn't disagree with the action to excuse them. I truly believed that they accidentally, possibly through no conscious action of their own, took a vitamin product called Super Charge, which contained among numerous ingredients ma-huang.

That still doesn't excuse the fact that they may have competed under the influence of a performance enhancing drug. Now, was that fair to the other competitors in the Trials? I think not. Remember, it's one thing to be excused for inadvertent use during competition, but whether excused or not, the individual still competed with a performance enhancing substance in his system. Did that make the difference? Did clean, drug-free athletes get cheated in the process?

A similar situation occurred in the 1988 Judo Olympic Trials when an athlete tested positive for ma-huang and it was considered inadvertent. To the Judo Federation's credit, though, it deemed that he had competed under the influence of a banned substance. Therefore, the federation, at some expense and difficulty, demanded a replay and brought the losing competitor and the positive athlete back to Colorado Springs for a re-qualifying competition. The positive athlete lost and was dropped from the Olympic Judo Team.

I think most rational people would agree with this approach, even though the outcome was unfortunate. The athlete who lost later admitted to me that although he was indeed unaware of the substance he took, he did feel considerably more hyped at the initial qualifying event than he did at the second competition in Colorado Springs.

I know there are difficult decisions for everyone involved: the sport bodies, the athletes, and all. Nonetheless, it's fair to the athletes that may have been cheated. Why didn't TAC consider this course of action for the occurrences in Indianapolis?

Well, that brings us back to the discussion of the inadvertent or innocent use clause. It just isn't fair to excuse the positive athlete on a technicality and, in the process, let him maintain his position on the team. Where is the appeal for the second- or third-place finisher? For the fourth-place finisher?

All this suggests a scenario that highlights this loophole in the testing process. Let's, for example, use the current rules for inadvertent use. Say Athlete Y has been through the testing process numerous times and knows the rules. He knows full well from all the educational lectures, the cautions at each testing episode, and the numerous publications available to remind him to beware of over-the-counter medications, vitamin supplements, and herbs. But this is the big event. The rules are such that you can be excused on a one-time-only basis. Therefore, now is the time to use the "gift"!

I can't tell you how many times I have advised not only the USOC Substance Abuse Committee, which governs the testing, but also USOC officials that this rule was not appropriate and was just another pitfall that would eventually hurt the program.

Another story shows how drug testing, or at least the threat of drug testing, can be used internationally as a tool for manipulating the competition: the "games behind the games," if you will. In 1986 the United States and the Soviet Union had the opportunity to compete against each other in a major multisport competition for the first time since the 1976 Olympic Summer Games in Montreal. The event: the Goodwill Games. The site: Moscow.

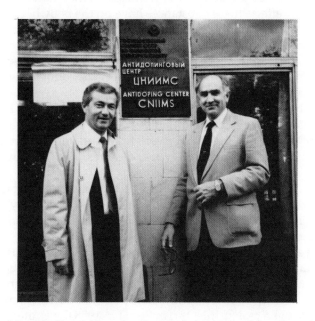

Dr. Voy and Dr. Catlin visiting the Soviet drug testing laboratory in Moscow.

Obviously, both countries were pretty geared up for this event. The word had traveled back to the American athletes before the Goodwill Games that there would indeed be drug testing, that all competitors would be subjected to after-competition drug tests. Accordingly, most athletes whom I knew confided in me that the Americans were getting off their drugs. They were stopping their anabolic-androgenic steroid cycles in time to have all these drugs clear their bodies, and they weren't planning on using any speed at the Games site.

What they found in Moscow, however, was something quite unexpected. There wasn't any drug testing. None. Evidently, the word the Americans had received about the testing for the 1986 Goodwill Games was a bogus rumor planted by someone with the precise intention of getting the Americans off their drugs.

Once the Americans found themselves halfway around the world without their drugs, it was too late to equal the competition. Many quickly noticed that some of the Eastern European athletes must have known there would be no drug testing because many appeared quite bulked up. The Europeans had continued their use of AAS right up to the Games. In addition, I would suspect they had no reservations about using various stimulants.

Thus, the Americans had been burned. Once they had stopped using their drugs, the effects these substances have on the body began to vanish. Other athletes, on the other hand, were physically *and chemically* primed for this competition. When the Games were over, the American delegation had been outclassed in almost every event, "proving" before the world for the first time in nearly a decade that the Soviet athletes were indeed the finest on earth.

Yet, it is the Soviet Union that boasts of having been the host nation for the first "drug-free" Olympic Games (the 1980 Olympic Games). After seeing their testing facilities in Moscow firsthand and after realizing the Soviets' willingness to play these types of games, I simply cannot believe that claim.

Hopefully, everyone will see that there are plenty of loopholes that can inhibit drug testing. Add to these loopholes the possibility of human manipulation of the testing process, and you can understand how drug testing poses little threat to many athletes.

There is yet one other way to avoid sanctions and disqualifications for doping violations: Sometimes national sport officials can actually talk an athlete out of trouble by lobbying their interests to the testing officials. It sounds ridiculous, I know. But believe it: I've seen it happen.

Few people even realize this, but in Seoul in 1988 the United States was in serious jeopardy of having one of its most visible teams disqualified. Evidently one of the American athletes competing tested positive for a high testosterone level. Because he was a member of a team, the whole team was subject to disqualification. U.S. officials, however, were somehow able to convince the IOC testing officials that the athlete in question had a natural testosterone ratio greater than 6:1—higher than any normal ratio I have ever seen personally.

So he got off the hook—not because he was *proven* innocent or because the IOC test could not prove his guilt beyond a doubt, but because of two other very important factors: He was American, and the American officials didn't want his team disqualified. You see, often it doesn't matter whether or not you're guilty as much as who you are and where you're from. I would suspect that if the athlete in question had been from Poland or Japan, the team would have been disqualified. Because his team was an Olympic power, though, he slipped by.

Incidentally, had this U.S. team been disqualified, it would have been the most controversial, scandalous story to be generated from the entire Seoul Olympiad, the Ben Johnson story notwithstanding.

Why do I now allege all these mysterious dealings? Because the athletes know that they happened. If athletes perceive this as truth and yet no one is willing to publicly discredit what has gone on in the past, nothing will change in the present or the future. Athletes will know claims that testing is fair and effective are lies. The predicament of taking the drugs and gambling in international competition will continue.

Surely there is need for reform. Getting to the bottom of all the past behavior is probably a hopeless task. Shouldn't we all admit to past problems and now commit ourselves to making sure that this alleged foul play won't or *can't* happen ever again?

Yes, there are ways to do this, and I'll tell you how later.

# 8

# The Road Not Taken

## *How Athletes Get Caught Up in the Drug Game*

Consider this. A number of elite-level athletes were asked if, hypothetically, they would be willing to take a special pill that would guarantee them an Olympic gold medal even if they knew this pill would kill them within a year. Over 50 percent of the athletes surveyed said yes.[23]

This is a terrifying indication of just how desperate athletes are to win. Some athletes are clearly willing to do anything in their attempts to earn the fame, glory, and wealth that come with winning. There are also many unethical physicians, trainers, and businessmen out there who are willing to cash in on this desperation. Is it any wonder, therefore, that the drug problem has reached such an enormous magnitude?

How, exactly, do athletes get involved with the dubious world of drug use? Unfortunately, such involvement is an easy process.

In the case of cocaine or marijuana, pushers, friends, or acquaintances may give a person the first taste of the drug. This may lead to a long, debilitating addiction—a problem that may arise from seemingly innocent, recreational origins, but one that will hamper the user for the rest of his or her life.

*Author's Note:* The IOC and the USOC do not ban the use of marijuana because they believe "marijuana is not considered a performance enhancing drug." I continue to disagree.

Marijuana is a major problem in sport because it is the gateway drug to other drug addictions, not least of all cocaine addiction. It is also used to enhance performance. The IOC and the USOC don't seem to appreciate the fact that through repeated use, marijuana can effectively allay apprehension and steady nerves in certain sports, just as do alcohol, tranquilizers, and beta-blockers. Through repeated use, the mind influencing, detrimental effects are tolerated, and the becalming and self-confidence effects can be used effectively by the individual. It's unfortunate, in my opinion, that this drug is not included in the list of banned drugs.

The process of addiction to other performance enhancing drugs, however, may be a bit different than the road athletes take to become involved with cocaine and marijuana. First, the desire to succeed, to be competitive, and to win is instilled in the minds of young people. The young athlete watching television sees an Olympian standing on the winner's podium to receive a gold medal, and the youngster thinks, "If only that could be me someday." Upon learning more about what really goes on in the local gyms and sport counterculture, the athlete quickly discovers the advantages gained from drugs.

Believe me, parents should not consider their aspiring young athlete sons and daughters naive when it comes to drug use. They are more sophisticated and knowledgeable than even most professionals and certainly the average parent. Those who think this is too general a statement are, in my opinion, the ones who are naive about drugs.

Sometimes, however, the young athlete needs a gentle nudge over the line by older and respected persons to get them to take the chance, to start using drugs. For example, perhaps the young athlete is a football player. He was a high school standout—indeed, good enough to earn the interest of college coaches. His dream is to play for State University, perhaps someday in the NFL.

A recruiting college football coach visits the athlete at his home and indicates that he wants to offer the young player a scholarship. The papers get signed, and the happy parents shake hands with the coach. On leaving, and possibly without realizing what effect his words have on the boy, the coach tells the athlete that he'd like to see him put on some weight before the fall camp begins. He might even suggest that by doing so, he will impress the other coaches and maybe see a little playing time. Therefore, it might be a good idea for him to bulk up a bit before camp.

Well, that's all that has to be said to get this kid's mind working and, in some cases, nudge him down the path toward anabolic-androgenic steroids. His parents, who are tickled to death that their son has gotten a scholarship, will then say, "Gee, the boy's only 185 pounds. He needs to gain 25, 30, 40 pounds more of lean muscle mass between June and August." It is absolutely impossible for that athlete to achieve his new goal in 2 to 3 months through weight training and good nutrition alone. The natural process, though certainly effective with more time, just won't get the quick job done. From that point, it will probably take only one trip to the local gym before this kid sees what others have done with drugs, which in turn points him directly toward anabolic-androgenic steroid use.

What we have here are the two key elements that lead to performance enhancing drug use: an incredible desire to succeed and the perceived impossibility of reaching a goal through normal, natural means. When these two situations present themselves to an athlete, desperation sets in. He has a seemingly impossible mission to accomplish and will then turn to whatever it takes to reach this objective. He may find the key to the dilemma, that is, a *supernatural* means to reach his goal—in this case, anabolic-androgenic steroids.

One can see how this problem might originate from innocent intentions. The coach wants to help the kid reach his goal. The athlete wants to do well. Sometimes, however, a user feels he or she has no other choice than to use drugs.

Perhaps the user will initially approach anabolic-androgenic steroids with the hope that one quick cycle will give him that 30-pound advantage by the time he arrives at football camp. What he doesn't realize at the time is that he has probably started the whole process of repeated use and addiction. Once the athlete enters his college campus and football camp at a svelte 235 pounds, he finds that he cannot let that image disappear during the season. One thing physicians do know about anabolic-androgenic steroids is that once you stop taking the drug, the gains made almost completely vanish. This individual wouldn't dare go back down to 185 pounds after enjoying his increased size and strength. Therein lies the basis for the psychological and physical addictions I have already described.

It is a very simple thing for coaches and sport officials to come out publicly in opposition to the use of performance enhancing steroids but then, on the basis of their demands on the athletes, force the athletes to take them. This isn't conscious coercion but a subconscious, almost subliminal suggestion that these athletes need to do something beyond their normal means to be the best they can be.

Now, this situation is a bit different elsewhere in the world. When government gets involved, the coerciveness of drug use isn't quite as subtle and, I suggest, is probably mandated. For example, in the 1970s and 1980s, if you were an East German athlete, we have been led to believe, the drug taking process was just part of their overall system.

In fact, recent accusations by former elite athletes in East Germany state that the East German Sport Federation actively promoted and regulated drug use among all East German athletes. Former world champion ski jumper Hans-Georg Aschenbach, who defected from East Germany in August 1988, and former East German Judo Federation Chairman Hans Juergen Noczenski, who defected in February 1989, told the West German newspaper *Bild Am Sonntag* in a July 1989 exposé that East German sport officials intimidated, manipulated, and advised their athletes into using performance enhancing drugs. Aschenbach and Noczenski both charged that all East German athletes were virtually force-fed performance enhancing drugs, beginning as early as age 13.

Among the athletes they named as users were 1988 Olympic figure skating champion Katarina Witt and six-time gold medalist in the Seoul swimming events Kristin Otto. Now that the East German border has opened, we're hearing more and more such accusations.

The question always comes up in these discussions as to why the Socialist countries, and East Germany in particular, produce such great athletes. Why isn't America number one in the world of sport? The answer has to do with two factors: national commitment and individual incentive on the part of the athletes. For example, East Germany, with 17 million people, made the commitment to be number one in a select group of sports. They supported their athletes from childhood to the grave, providing them with the very best facilities, training techniques, and sports medicine and science. All of these resources are housed in the Leipzig Institute. The Soviets, of course, have their Institute of Physical Culture. The United States has nothing even close, the Colorado Springs Olympic Training Center notwithstanding.

More importantly, given such a commitment, East German and Soviet athletes are their countries' elite. Their Saturday morning cartoon doesn't feature Superman but a robust, good-looking athlete who grows up in sport, wins an Olympic medal, makes the transition from sport into military service, and as a national hero motivates and educates young people to live healthy and fit lives. This character is also the prime motivator behind the movement to curtail smoking and drinking and stop drug use.

The individual rewards for the Socialist sports hero are not just the automobile and a better flat for his or her parents to live in but the ability to travel outside the country.

---

*Author's Note:*   For the purpose of this discussion, I am describing the East German travel incentive that preceded the sweeping reforms enacted in the DDR in late 1989.

---

The average East German or Soviet athlete may have dedicated his or her life to sport for the chance to compete in a place like Kansas City and come home with a medal and a pair of blue jeans, something previously unavailable to the ordinary citizen in Moscow or Dresden. It's as simple as that. Drug use during training, and whatever else the coaches or officials deem necessary to excel, was part of the bargain. The athlete didn't worry about where, how much, or what side effects would result from the training regimen that included drug use. You will remember the East German jubilation that followed the dismantling of the Berlin Wall: Before 1989 only the athletes tasted such freedom. Thus, from the images we see on television today, we have begun to see how enormously powerful this freedom incentive was.

---

*Author's Note:*   Recently we've begun to hear that East German athletes were not idolized by the public but were actually resented for receiving this preferential treatment.

---

Now, I'm not saying we should offer proportionately magnificent incentives to our developing athletes. No way—we have a different culture and ethic. However, there is a way for the United States to upgrade its international sport status, to provide a better opportunity and lifestyle for our elite athletes, and to create some needed incentives—but only if the United States wishes to make the commitment. I'll have more to say on that line in chapter 9.

Naturally, the East Germans have disputed these recurring accusations of past drug use, saying that it is all merely slanderous propaganda. In fact, the East Germans even seem to be talking about more involvement in the international antidoping movement than ever before.

Many of my American athlete contacts, though, are already saying that we should not trust the Soviets or East Germans to abide by any agreement. These Americans aren't worried about out-of-competition testing themselves, either. Some say they will try to train without AAS, but if their times increase they will go back on AAS. Several have already indicated they have an inside source in The Athletics Congress (TAC) who tells them when to expect testing. This is a point in my favor as I continuously implore the sport community to allow testing to be done by an independent agency.

If the East Germans did drugs, they did them effectively. Few, if any, got caught, and the programs worked because the athletes were in the hands of specialists.

To an American, buying and correctly using performance enhancing drugs is much more problematic. Because the IOC and the USOC have banned certain performance enhancing drugs and because such drug use is considered unethical by most physicians and sports officials, Western athletes are forced to find more dubious sources for their drugs, namely, the black market. They turn to the black market in their attempt to remain competitive with athletes from countries like the Soviet Union. Unfortunately, dealing with the black market can be a deadly game.

Once athletes feel a desperate desire to succeed and once they feel they have no place to turn for help, they might tell their friends of the problem they are facing. Perhaps they will go down to their local gyms and tell their workout partners. Whatever the case, sooner or later they are bound to bump into someone who can point them in the direction of anabolic-androgenic steroids. In almost any local gym, particularly body building gyms, there are usually many individuals who can provide free access to knowledge on steroid programs. Quite often these gurus provide free access to the drugs themselves.

If athletes really want to buy anabolic-androgenic steroids, all they would really have to do is go down to a bodybuilding gym, meet the right people, and express interest in purchasing drugs; they would be well on their way to buying them. It wouldn't matter if they were in Los Angeles, California, Doylestown, Pennsylvania, or Boise, Idaho. These drugs can be bought anywhere.

In working on this book, I had an assistant go out and try to purchase anabolic-androgenic steroids in order to test this theory. How long did it take him to find these drugs? Only a walk into a gym. After a 10-minute conversation, he was handed an order form, went to the nearest phone, and for 25 cents placed an order that he received in the mail in 6 days.

Just how do anabolic-androgenic steroid distributors get these drugs? The black market for AAS, as I have said, is quite large and prosperous. Authorities estimate this to be a $200 million business, and growing.

I think the best way to describe how the black market operates would be to describe a real-life situation. Several years ago United States Customs authorities cracked down on what was believed to be the largest anabolic-androgenic steroid smuggling operation in North America. The investigation that has resulted from this bust has given drug control authorities a clearer picture of how the black market operates.

Former British Olympian David Jenkins, who anchored Britain's 4 × 400-meter relay to a silver medal in the 1972 Olympic Games in Munich, was imprisoned in California. After his competitive career was over, Jenkins remained active in the world of athletics as the mastermind of a massive anabolic-androgenic steroid operation based in San Diego, California. At the time of Jenkin's arrest, Phillip Halpern, the U.S. District Attorney in San Diego, estimated that Jenkin's operation controlled 70 percent of the illegal wholesale anabolic-androgenic steroid sales in the United States.

His operation was centered around San Diego and Tijuana, Mexico. Tijuana is a free trade zone; thus, the sale of pharmaceutical products there is not illegal. Jenkins hooked up with a pharmaceutical manufacturer and importer in Tijuana called Labratorios Milano. Labratorios Milano supplied the anabolic-androgenic steroids, and Jenkins sold them under the name of United Pharmaceuticals from the Fiesta Americana Hotel in Tijuana.

In most cases, an American anabolic-androgenic steroid dealer would cross the border to work with Jenkins. After handing Jenkins the required payment for his supply, this dealer would be instructed by Jenkins to go to a designated spot, usually a motel back in the United States, where the shipment could be delivered.

Jenkins had men working for him who would smuggle these drugs across the U.S. border and through the customs checkpoint on a daily basis. One former Jenkins employee admitted to crossing the border with anabolic-androgenic steroids hidden on his body, or in parts of his car, three times daily, 7 days a week, for a period of 6 months. Once the drugs were inside the United States, they would be loaded into a truck and left at the delivery point for the buyer to pick up. The buyer, having paid Jenkins in Mexico, could then drive away with his truckload of anabolic-androgenic steroids back to his gym or spa, where he would in turn sell them to his athlete customers.

It is important to remember that in Tijuana the sale of these drugs is not illegal. Possession of anabolic-androgenic steroids on a doctor's prescription is also not illegal in the United States. But smuggling these drugs into the United States for resale is indeed illegal, and this is where Jenkins ran afoul of the law.

Tony Fitton, also known as Dr. Hormone, ran a successful drug importation business in Albuquerque, New Mexico, until federal agents finally caught up to him. He served nearly 1 year in prison. Interestingly, after he was released, he was approached by Jenkins, who was looking for a business partner, but Fitton refused.

In an interview for a recent BBC program titled "Dying to Win," which detailed the Jenkins operation, Fitton admitted that if the public knew who some of his customers were, they would be quite surprised.

Sometimes, buying anabolic-androgenic steroids can be as easy as picking up a muscle magazine and sending off an order form by mail. Often, foreign anabolic-androgenic steroid distribution houses like Jenkins's company place classified advertisements in muscle magazines soliciting orders for these drugs. Today all an interested customer needs to do is acquire an order form, send off some cash, and his drugs will be home-delivered in a matter of a few weeks.

In an effort to stop this problem, Senator Joseph Biden of Delaware has introduced a federal bill that would prohibit the sale and distribution of performance enhancing drugs by mail. In another attempt to crack down on the anabolic-androgenic steroid black market, California State Representative Mel Levine has introduced a bill that would put the illegal distribution of anabolic-androgenic steroids in the same controlled substance classification as cocaine. A draft copy of Levine's bill would define 24 types of anabolic-androgenic steroids under Category II of the Controlled Substances Act.

But there are other places where athletes can find these drugs. Sometimes an athlete might find his own coach to be a performance enhancing drug guru. Many sports fans have heard of Charlie Francis, Ben Johnson's coach and guru. Francis made Johnson the fastest man in the world, as he made sprinter Angella Taylor Issajenko one of the fastest women in the world.

Johnson's story is truly a rags-to-riches (-to-rags) story. He arrived in Canada from his poor homeland of Jamaica as a scrawny young boy. At the age of 15, he began working with Francis. Over the course of the next 11 years, Francis built Johnson into the most formidable sprinter in the world.

The problem was, Francis used anabolic-androgenic steroids to make Johnson the athlete he became. In the 1988 Seoul Olympic Games, Johnson was disqualified when traces of an anabolic-androgenic steroid appeared in his urine sample after he had crushed the world record in the 100-meter dash by running a time of 9.79 seconds. The rest, so they say, is history.

The Canadian government opened an inquiry—called the Dubin Inquiry because it was led by Charles Dubin, the associate chief justice of Ontario—into drug abuse in sport, particularly the Ben Johnson situation. According to testimony by Johnson, Francis gave him anabolic-androgenic steroids for the first time in 1981. Johnson said that he wasn't exactly sure what he was taking at the time, but in subsequent months it became clear to him that he was using banned substances.

The real key to this issue, in my mind, is the absolute blind trust that Johnson had in his coach and Dr. Jamie Astaphan, who served as medical advisor, confidant, and source of drugs for Francis and his athletes. Whether Johnson knew of the potential dangers of drug use, or the potential for being caught, may never be fully resolved. Johnson's comments indicate that he was not as well informed about the possible side effects of these drugs as he could have been. Astaphan and Francis, on the other hand, contend that Johnson was well aware of the business he was dealing in.

Either way, we do know that Johnson was willing to follow every instruction his physician and his coach gave him—to a T. And why not? They were the men who were making his dreams come true. Through Francis and Astaphan, Johnson had achieved stature, fame, and considerable wealth. An Associated Press wire story quoted Johnson at the Dubin Inquiry: "I'm not the coach. I just take orders. . . . My concern is to concentrate on just [running]. . . . Nobody took time out to tell me what the side effects were. But I was making all this money, so. . . ."

In short, someone who wanted to train for Francis had to do whatever it took to win. The athlete had to want to do everything possible to reach the top. Part of the coach-athlete relationship in this case involved taking anabolic-androgenic steroids. Just like an extra few laps around the track or an extra hour in the weight room, drug use was considered an integral

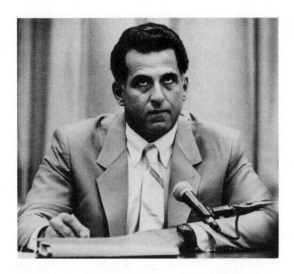

Dr. Jamie Astaphan testifying at the Dubin Inquiry.
*Note.* © Allsport USA. 1989. Reprinted by permission.

part of the overall training process. Someone who trusted the coach, which would be true if the coach had brought him or her from nothing to the world championship, would follow the coach's every order.

This attitude is a key reason I don't like to condemn the athletes themselves. I just don't think they're completely at fault, particularly when they are simply following orders. Though in most cases they realize they are cheating, they regard it as a necessary evil if they are to remain competitive. Besides, many of them realize that a significant number of their competition are using drugs as well. So who's to blame them? I say if there are any fingers to be pointed, they should be aimed at the coaches and doctors who are advising the athletes to use drugs and at the sport officials who allow an unfair system to exist. In the drug abuse rehabilitation business, we call these people enablers.

Canada is not the only place where coaches get their own athletes hooked on drugs. There are many coaches with similar attitudes toward drug use working right here in the United States. Chuck DeBus of Santa Monica, California, has built a reputation for sending this message to many of his athletes: If you don't want to use drugs, I don't want to work with you.

DeBus was the model for the nasty, overbearing coach in the 1982 film *Personal Best*. He has coached many national level athletes, including former U.S. sprint champion Diane Williams. In an April 1989 Senate inquiry into drug abuse in sport, Williams charged that DeBus had coerced her into using anabolic-androgenic steroids while she was training under him in the early 1980s.[24] As reported in the April 4, 1989, *USA Today*, Williams said, "I trusted a coach who had no interest in me as a person."[25] According to Williams, DeBus cared only about winning, and winning at all costs.

Williams subsequently stopped her use of anabolic-androgenic steroids when she began suffering several side effects, including facial hair growth, deepened voice, and severe depression.

I have heard similar stories from other athletes who have worked under DeBus. For example, a javelin thrower who once trained under DeBus, Marilyn B. White, wrote me this account:

> I was approached on numerous occasions by one of my former coaches, Chuck DeBus, to begin a training program that included the daily use of steroids. I was attending California State University, Northridge, at the time [fall 1977–spring 1978]. Along with his suggestion, Mr. DeBus stated that I would never be good enough to become a national contender unless I were to take steroids. I declined, my decision based on my feelings that if that is what it takes to become the "elite," then I did not care to be any part of track and field competition. I also did not feel that the benefits outweighed the health risks. I eventually withdrew from competition, even though I had the great potential to become a national and world calibre javelin thrower, feeling that I was at a distinct disadvantage in competing against other national calibre athletes whose training regimen included the use of anabolic steroids.

Clearly, we have to crack down on coaches who are controlled by a "win at all costs" attitude, who are willing to treat their young athletes like pieces of meat, and who scoff at the concept of fairness in sport. If these individuals don't care about the health, the emotional welfare, and the personal development of the athletes they work with, and if they don't care for the concept of integrity and fairness in sport, what business do they have being coaches?

The Athletics Congress, which governs track and field in the United States, conducted an investigation of Chuck DeBus's dubious practices—after delaying his hearing seven times! In the fall of 1989 TAC vowed to rid track and field of drugs, and promised it was going to bring this issue to light. TAC vowed that if DeBus was guilty of infractions, as dozens of his former athletes have alleged, it would come down hard on him.

But what TAC said and what TAC did are two different things. In fact, at one point the two parties seemed to have reached an out-of-inquiry agreement. TAC announced that it had handed DeBus a 2-year suspension from coaching. DeBus had agreed to the suspension on the stipulation that he did not have to make any admission of guilt. After facing considerable opposition to this weak solution, TAC reopened the investigation, but closed it to the media. Finally, TAC announced that DeBus had been suspended for life. On July 17, 1990, *USA Today* reported that DeBus would appeal to TAC to reverse its ruling.[26] I hope TAC will remain firm in its decision, but even if TAC does decide to make an example of DeBus, it will have done nothing to address the depth of this problem among hundreds of coaches. On the other hand, if TAC reverses its ruling and lets DeBus go with a slap on the hand, it will have provided yet one more clear demonstration of the hypocrisy prevalent in its effort to stop drug abuse among athletes.

There are other sources athletes have to acquire anabolic-androgenic steroids if they aren't buying them on the black market or being advised directly by a coach on this issue. Concerned coaches need to know this. Sadly, there are a great number of physicians out there who are willing to provide athletes with prescriptions for performance enhancing drugs.

Perhaps none of them had a more dubious reputation for being a steroid guru than Robert B. Kerr, MD, of San Gabriel, California. Dr. Kerr, the subject of a 1985 CBS "60 Minutes" interview, was considered to be one of the most reliable sources American athletes had for anabolic-androgenic steroids in the years leading up to 1985. Many of Dr. Kerr's patients were the United States' finest track-and-field athletes. Indeed, if the general public saw some of the faces in his waiting room at that time, it probably would have recognized many. By 1985 Dr. Kerr estimated his anabolic-androgenic steroid–using patient total to be nearly 3,000, though many contend this is a very conservative estimate.

The process for receiving anabolic-androgenic steroids directly from Dr. Kerr involved the price of an office (consultation) visit, where he would discuss the potential side effects of AAS use. Having received the necessary informed consent and learned what the athlete wanted to use the drug for, he would then, in most cases, provide the necessary prescription.

Also, Dr. Kerr had published a book in 1982 titled *The Practical Use of Anabolic Steroids With Athletes* (now out of print), which discussed the various benefits (and dangers) that could be realized through anabolic-androgenic steroid use.

Now, one might think that I would find a lot of fault with Dr. Kerr. I basically don't. In fact, we are friends. Dr. Kerr and I simply had a very major split in medical philosophy. He became the "steroid doctor" prior to all the current controversy and before the official IOC and USOC bans. As Dr. Kerr has testified before the Dubin Inquiry, after realizing 4 years ago that the athletes were using doses far in excess of his recommendations and were stacking and fooling with growth hormone, he stopped prescribing the drugs.

Providing athletes with anabolic-androgenic steroids during the early years was something that a great many doctors did. They felt that because it wasn't illegal, their ethical basis for meeting the athletes' demands was established. One way or another, athletes were bound to get involved with anabolic-androgenic steroids once they broke into the elite level of their sport; it was general knowledge that most elite athletes were using performance enhancing drugs of one form or another. Dr. Kerr and others thought that athletes should at least take the drugs under the care and supervision of a qualified physician. Should any adverse side effects occur, at least they would receive medical attention and not be allowed to get into more trouble.

I, too, experienced the same pressures from athletes to prescribe the drugs. My philosophy, however, was and still is that a physician should do no harm and that giving drugs intended for therapy where no therapeutic need existed was wrong. Now, after I've developed a deeper understanding of fair competition and the potential health risks, I think my professional philosophy was and is the correct one. I think a lot of doctors involved at the time, including Dr. Kerr, have since changed their ways.

Times change and we learn from our mistakes. Today there are 25 states that have enacted laws or promulgated stricter regulations dealing with prescribing AAS. Most of these regulations make it unethical practice for physicians to prescribe AAS to athletes for performance enhancement purposes. Of these 25 states, 9—Oklahoma, California, Florida, Idaho, Kansas, Minnesota, North Carolina, Texas, and Utah—have placed AAS under state controlled-substance acts that make it a felony to prescribe AAS for nontherapeutic purposes. I hope others will follow. Possibly AAS will ultimately fall under Category II of the federal Controlled Substances Act.

The professional logic, that with medical supervision these drugs can be used safely, just doesn't fly. Some doctors have to learn the hard way. "I really thought [supervising AAS use] was one way we could get them away from the black market, from the high doses and from using the multiple types of steroids," Dr. Kerr admitted in a 1989 USA Today interview. "But I learned I simply can't trust these [athletes]."[27]

I think Dr. Kerr got involved with the drug scene because he cared about athletes. But there are other doctors in this world whose motives are less altruistic and whose methods are simply sadistic, in my opinion. One of the world's most celebrated drug gurus is West German Professor Armin Klümper. Known as one of the foremost father figures in German sports medicine circles, Klümper is also nicknamed Mr. Syringe.

In 1987 I became aware of one of the most incredible stories regarding multiple drug use, legal and illegal, that I had ever come across. I want to relate to you a synopsis of this tragedy because it describes the magnitude of the problem we face in stemming the tide of drug abuse in sport. It is also a clear example of how blindly athletes will trust drug gurus, in this case Klümper, to help them achieve fame and stature. This story was reported in the West German magazine *Der Spiegel* on September 7, 1987.

West German heptathlete Birgit Dressel, age 26, died on April 10, 1987. During her last year, Dressel had become a world contender, rising from 33rd to 6th place in the world rankings. She had substantially increased her muscle development and her endurance.

Each day for a year before her death, Dressel swallowed her usual diet pills, tablets, and capsules, a total of nine in all. These pills included medications doctors usually give to treat aging diseases, such as arteriosclerosis, swelling of the legs, allergies, osteoporosis, inflammation of the intestines, arterial cramps, and dropsy. Some of these drugs were scientifically effective, but many others were unproven.[28] Besides these pills that Klümper gave her, Dressel also took Stromba, a.k.a. stanozolol, an anabolic-androgenic steroid she obtained from another physician. In her last year, Dressel had taken over 400 injections of 40 different medications, including some harmless substances such as bee pollen and various homeopathic medicines.

On the day Dressel first complained of pain, she went to see Mr. Syringe, who proceeded to inject her backside numerous times with Ney-Dop, a mixture of "standardized macromolecules of fresh cells from animal brain and placenta." After 3 days of unbearable pain, Dressel died. The cause of Birgit Dressel's death was listed as an acute allergic reaction, oversensitivity and a breakdown of her body's resistance to the hundreds of medicines she had subjected herself to over the course of her last year. The public prosecutor found Mr. Syringe to be innocent for lack of proof of negligent or harmful conduct.

In many cases, athletes do not need to turn to doctors, coaches, or black market sources to find performance enhancing drugs. Often, athletes can get hold of these substances from other athletes with whom they are training. This type of stuff happened (and probably still happens) right inside the very walls of the United States Olympic Training Center in Colorado Springs.

Take the case of female cyclist Cindy Olavarri. Olavarri, who lives in Oakland, California, was the model natural athlete in the late 1970s and early 1980s. She was a gifted performer, and there were few sports she couldn't do well. She took up competitive cycling at the age of 22, and she quickly ascended to the ranks of the national elite.

By the time she turned 26, however, Olavarri reached a plateau in her career. She grew frustrated with her performances and realized that she needed to take some drastic measures if she wanted to truly achieve world-class stature.

So Olavarri began taking anabolic-androgenic steroids. She was given these drugs, and instructions for how she should use them, by fellow athletes while she was training at the Olympic Training Center. Olavarri used anabolic-androgenic steroids off and on for the next 3 years, and her career once again began to climb steadily upward. In the 1984 Olympic Trials, Olavarri earned a position on the United States Cycling Team.

But she was found positive for anabolic-androgenic steroid use by the after-competition drug testing at the Trials. She was then privately kicked off the team, an event that Olavarri admits shattered her hopes and dreams. What followed were several years of various drug addictions, including amphetamines and other stimulants and depressants.

Today, however, Olavarri is realizing perhaps the greatest tragedy associated with her use of addicting drugs. She has experienced liver damage, she now has complicated allergic reactions to foods she had never been allergic to before, and almost every joint in her body aches. Olavarri can now ride her bike only two or three times a week, providing she takes it easy, a sad condition for a woman who became one of the world's top cyclists in only 4 years.

Olavarri has, however, channeled these problems into positive action. Today she works by visiting young children and speaking—using her own story as a prime example—about the dangers of drug abuse.

So many parents, coaches, and athletic colleagues are shocked when they hear such horror stories. They wonder where they went wrong by not becoming aware of the problem. Often they want to learn about drug abuse and how to recognize someone who is using drugs or how people become addicted. Other than actually catching someone in the act, most people are too naive to pick up the telltale signs.

There are several key signs that can sometimes give a drug user away. I have found the characteristics listed in the box to be quite common among frequent drug users. A parent, coach, or friend who recognizes these signs should confront the individual with their suspicions. Also, it's never too soon to suggest professional help. The sooner drug users are found out, the greater the chance for treatment success. Sometimes, in my experience, the user is almost subliminally looking to be busted; that is frequently the easiest way to shake off peer influences with no loss of "honor."

The stories of athletes like Birgit Dressel are ones of polypharmacy that result from looking for shortcuts to gain the competitive edge. They usually begin innocently when an athlete takes a vitamin or a supplement. Once the mind-set is established that something extra is needed, the problem grows. Discovery of the performance enhancing drug effect of stimulants and anabolic-androgenic steroids follows. The athlete sees that these drugs work; from then on, a pattern is established of chasing after that fountain of athletic prowess, or shortcut to success. Athletes are driven to allow gurus, scientists, and physicians to do almost anything or give them almost any substance without thought of the possible consequences.

There does not seem to be enough emphasis on ethics in controlling certain physicians and scientists who are willing to take advantage of athletes to enhance their own reputations and careers. There should be.

## COMMON CHARACTERISTICS
## OF FREQUENT DRUG USERS

- Mood swings from sullen and withdrawn to oversensitive, easily provoked, irritable, less affectionate, uncooperative, hostile, and secretive—especially on the phone

- Loss of interest in school sport or practice

- New, peculiar circle of friends

- Increasing tardiness or absence from work, school, or practice

- Considerable weight loss in a short time

- Always needing money

- Avoiding home responsibilities

- Not responding to family and friends in a usual or expected way

- Change of dress style or interests

- Refusing to discuss friends; strongly defensive about any negative talk concerning drug issues

- Mental deterioration; heightened sensitivity to touch, smell, and taste

- Sudden change of appetite; either no appetite or excessive appetite

- Paranoid behavior

# 9

# The Money Pot

## The Politics That Control the United States Olympic Committee

One of the hot questions of the day seems to be, ''Why isn't the United States the Olympic power it once was?''

In other words, people want to know why the richest nation in the world (in terms of combined financial and human resources) is gradually becoming a second-rate world sports power.

Good question.

This question has been floating around amateur sports circles in the United States for some time now. Some people like to answer the question with this: ''Oh, those Russians are all using steroids. We'll never beat them because they're cheating.''

Sure, some Eastern European athletes have used drugs to enhance their performances for years. But so have some Americans. Thus, I don't believe drugs alone are the issue here. The East Germans and the Soviets aren't using drugs to gain the competitive edge on the Americans, at least not with drugs many Americans aren't also using.

The Eastern Europeans, however, are using drugs more effectively than we are. They have the science of performance enhancement mastered. Their athletes aren't using black market drugs or working under the guidance of steroid gurus. The Eastern Europeans are working with experts.

Perhaps this accounts for some advantage on the playing field, but I don't think it's the real reason for the difference in performance levels. I think much of our slip in international sports stature has to do with the ineffectiveness of the very system our nation relies on to develop our young athletes.

In my opinion, much of the blame for the American decline in sport worldwide should be placed on the shoulders of one organization: my former employer, the United States Olympic Committee (USOC).

While working inside the five rings at the Olympic Training Center in Colorado Springs, I learned that the USOC is, to many, nothing more than a "money pot." Our Olympic movement is fueled by the generous financial support of corporate America. Indeed, the various Olympic sponsors pour millions and millions of dollars into the USOC money pot with the intention of enhancing the American Olympic effort. Unfortunately, often that money is swallowed up by USOC overhead, and precious little finds its way to those whom the financial backing of corporate America could most significantly benefit, the athletes.

New programs, new ideas must be developed, but, contrary to what some USOC executives might believe, I don't think this calls for drumming more funds out of corporations or the American government. In my mind, the money is already there. It just shouldn't be wasted. The USOC has to do a better job of controlling and spending funds.

Historically, the USOC, which was established in 1896, was only an international sports "travel agency." Based in a small office in New York City, the USOC had the main responsibility to coordinate the assemblage of our Olympic Team and see to it that these athletes made it to the Olympic Games. The USOC also served as a liaison between American athletes and the International Olympic Committee (IOC). In terms of directing athletic policy and coordinating grassroots sports programs in the United States, however, the USOC was a relative nonentity.

For the most part, the job of training athletes, organizing amateur sport programs, coordinating competitions, and implementing sport policy was divided between two powerful organizations, the Amateur Athletic Union (AAU) and the National Collegiate Athletic Association (NCAA). These two organizations often feuded, causing a quasi-power struggle within the world of American amateur sport. Consequently, after the United States had been outgunned by the East Germans and the Soviets in the 1976 Olympic Summer Games in Montreal (the first stages of its decline in international athletic dominance), this power struggle garnered much deserved attention.

In 1976 the United States government decided to look at the American amateur sports system. A study was conducted by the President's Commission on Olympic Sports appointed by President Gerald Ford. Its purpose was to examine and remedy the situation by suggesting more efficient means to control the United States' Olympic movement.

The result of the Commission's work was Public Law 95-606, also known as the Amateur Sports Act of 1978, passed by the Ninety-fifth Congress of the United States. The Amateur Sports Act designated the United States Olympic Committee the coordinating body responsible for selecting the

U.S. Olympic Team and arranging for its participation in the Games. Also created by the Amateur Sports Act were a number of vertically integrated national governing bodies (NGBs), such as The Athletics Congress (TAC), U.S. Swimming, Inc. (USS), and the USA Amateur Boxing Federation (USA/ABF). These NGBs were given more power to govern their own sports individually, coordinating national competitions and so on under the guidance of their respective international federations.

The move effectively shifted the power base from two organizations (the AAU and the NCAA) to one all-powerful governing body (the USOC) and a number of other smaller confederations of sport (the NGBs, of which there are 41). That is the system we still have. In essence, the model is similar to the United States governmental system. The USOC, the central power, is equal in relative stature to the federal government. Each NGB, which has more direct influence over the day-to-day affairs within its own sport, is like a powerful state government that has its own international relations responsibilities.

When Congress passed the Amateur Sports Act of 1978, it did not appropriate any funding for the USOC, though the Commission advised that it would take a one-time infusion of $215 million and annual funding of $83 million to make the U.S. competitive. What the USOC did get, however, was a new home. The city of Colorado Springs, Colorado, made 36 acres of land and some old postwar government office buildings available to the USOC, and the USOC gladly accepted. So we had a new Olympic headquarters and a blueprint for operation.

The job of paying for this organization, though, was the first major task of the USOC hierarchy. The USOC had to quickly evolve into a big business. Believe me, today the amateur sports business in the United States is *big* business. Any doubters of this simply have to realize that the NCAA earns literally billions of dollars by selling television rights for basketball and football games alone. The USOC and NGBs earn millions of dollars from sponsorships and TV rights every year.

The USOC power structure is difficult to understand, for this organization is probably one of the most complicated bureaucracies on earth. At the top is the president, who today is Robert H. Helmick, Esq., of Des Moines, Iowa. He is one of the six top USOC officers, who are all volunteers: They aren't paid by the USOC, and they don't work in Colorado Springs. Joining the president as USOC officers are vice presidents William B. Tutt, George M. Steinbrenner III, and Michael Lenard, Esq.; secretary Charles U. Foster; and treasurer Leroy T. Walker, PhD.

Under the USOC officers is the Executive Committee, which is composed of 16 members including the officers, and is chaired by the president. All members of this committee are also volunteers. They meet approximately six times each year to establish protocol for supervision of the daily affairs of the USOC and enact policies created by the third branch of the USOC, the Executive Board. The rest of the year, they tend to their normal jobs throughout the country.

The Executive Board is the real power base when it comes to directing policy for USOC financial affairs and programming. This Board is made up of approximately 97 members—again, all volunteers—who meet three times every year. Prior to 1990 there was also a House of Delegates, made up of over 300 members who met annually, which had the authority to elect officers and to amend or repeal the USOC constitution and bylaws. The House of Delegates really did nothing more, however, than spend enormous amounts of money to fly its members to the annual convention. The Executive Committee recommended that the House of Delegates be disbanded after its February 1990 meeting, yielding its powers to an expanded Executive Board. That was a good move.

The USOC headquarters in Colorado Springs is called the Olympic House. The Olympic House is where all full-time, salaried staff members, from secretaries to fund-raising executives to the executive director, work.

The Olympic House is run by the executive director or secretary general, who is at this time Harvey Schiller (replacing Baaron Pittenger in late 1989). The Olympic House staff controls the day-to-day, nuts-and-bolts operation of the United States Olympic movement. They are, however, directly supervised and controlled by the USOC volunteer officers and the Executive Committee. The staff never dictates policy.

The staffs of the Olympic Training Center and of Sports Medicine and Science have their own offices on the Center Campus in Colorado Springs. The Center for Sports Medicine and Science, located on the grounds of the actual Training Center, was my home base when I was working with the USOC. For a complete visual understanding of the USOC structure, see Figure 4.

So what are the problems with the USOC? First of all, it is too big. A common expression tells that too many cooks spoil the broth. Well, that is certainly the case with the USOC. In addition to the officers, the Executive Committee, and the Board of Directors, there are some 21 volunteer advisory committees. Each committee meets two or three times per year, each member receiving free transportation, housing, and per diem subsidy. All total, there are over 150 individuals operating on the periphery and in the dark as to the mission of the USOC. An interesting note here is that in my 5 years of service, at least three concerted efforts were made by officers and staff to develop a mission statement for the USOC. One was never defined. Unlike most successful corporate organizations, the USOC certainly does not appear to be goal oriented.

Seldom do the committee members have hands-on experience or day-to-day working knowledge of what actually goes on at the Training Centers of global USOC-sponsored programs. The only direct work with athletes occurs at the Training Center and with the sports medicine staff. Yet, these

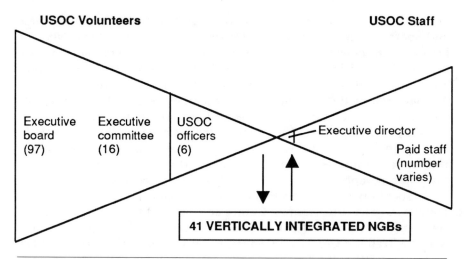

**USOC Volunteers**                                    **USOC Staff**

Executive board (97) | Executive committee (16) | USOC officers (6)

Executive director

Paid staff (number varies)

**41 VERTICALLY INTEGRATED NGBs**

**Figure 4.**   USOC organizational structure. *Note.* The NGBs control the majority of the vote of the executive board.

paid staff members, who work in the trenches every day with the athletes, are hand-bound and relatively powerless, in terms of the overall strategy/ decision-making process; they do not make any independent policy decisions whatsoever. Nothing gets done in the USOC without the Executive Board's seal of approval. This is difficult to come by, considering the fact that a 90-member volunteer governing body must agree on a given policy. Moreover, this group only meets three times each year. So nothing—I mean *nothing*—gets done quickly in the USOC.

Unfortunately, various departments of the USOC seem rather inept at communicating with each other, even within the very boundaries of the Training Center. For example, in my opinion, the administrative staff (the Olympic House staff) and the Executive Committee know very little about what goes on at the Training Center or Sports Medicine and Science facilities. In turn, the Training Center staff is not well aware of what's happening inside Olympic House.

In my personal experience as head of the Division of Sports Medicine and Science, I gathered that former Executive Director Col. F. Don Miller had a good working knowledge of our operation but never had to involve himself directly. His successor, Gen. George Miller, had sincerely attempted to understand the everyday workings of the entire operation.

However, while I was there, the executive officers and most other Olympic House staff members rarely visited the sports medicine facilities except to get a curbstone medical diagnosis or advice. They rarely ventured out of Olympic House and across the quadrangle except to get a bargain-priced meal at the athletes' dining hall. Thus, in my opinion, they had very little understanding of the services provided by the Training Center and Sports Medicine and Science Department. This lack of involvement hampered the effectiveness of the USOC as a whole when it came to making credible decisions about Training Center operations or drug testing and sports medicine. For example, most decisions relative to the white elephant Marquette, Michigan, Training Center were made by the volunteers without Training Center director Larry McCollum's advice.

I was personally irritated when the individuals in Olympic House, lacking any understanding of what we in Sports Medicine and Science could provide to the athletes, constantly complained about the money we spent. They had no appreciation for the fact that their job was to raise funds to be spent on the athletes. Every nickel I spent at the USOC was on athletes. In fact, the Training Center and Sports Medicine and Science really offered some of the only direct services available to the athletes. Yet, the Training Center and Sports Medicine budgets together added up to only a little over 20 percent of the total USOC budget. That's a small amount of the pot to be given to the focal point of the organization, the athletes.

The USOC made great strides under the leadership of former President William Simon and Executive Director F. Don Miller. Today, however, I see a huge obstruction to progress in the form of a conflict between the professional staff and the volunteers. This is a major issue, and it is tearing the organization down like a cancer that is malignant and may, in my opinion, ultimately be terminal.

While I worked for the USOC, we experienced four major changes in the executive director position, most due to personality conflicts with the USOC officers. The 1987 dismissal of former Secretary General George Miller was the most blatant example of this conflict. In my opinion, there hasn't been anyone better qualified to run the organization than Gen. Miller. But, according to Miller, the USOC officers got rid of him for one simple reason: The president couldn't get along with him.

The Olympic cause is always bigger than the individual, as it should be. However, too many good leaders have been lost to the Olympic movement for the sake of preserving several men's egos. A real shame here is that the high turnover of USOC staff members in recent years has cost the USOC millions of dollars, money that could have been spent on athletes. For example, it cost the USOC approximately $1 million to fire Gen. Miller and former USOC lobbyist/public relations expert Gen. Dick Abel and buy out the remaining terms of their contracts.

These men were also working on significant fund-raising projects when they were shown the door, projects such as the Olympic coin project and federal tax check-off legislation to benefit to the USOC. When these men were let go, their programs stagnated or died altogether. In particular, the coin program never got off and running in time to contribute effectively to the fund-raising effort before the 1988 Games.

Thus, the long-term ramifications of firing Gen. Miller and Gen. Abel became devastating. Some estimate this managerial blunder ultimately cost the USOC 15 to 25 million dollars in lost revenues, all because the president didn't like somebody. (I'll describe this situation more later on.)

In years gone by, the job of watching over amateur sports competitions was accepted and graciously performed by royalty. Remember, it was the elite class—the barons and dukes, and even the princes and princesses of the world—who started the whole ball rolling when the modern Olympic format was established in the late 19th century. And the reason for this was simple. These individuals did not *need* sport in any way. Their motives were basically altruistic, though it might be argued that being involved with the Olympic Games certainly did not hurt their images. These people were the ideal administrators for the Olympic movement because they were usually well traveled, diplomatic, and well schooled. They had a wealth of ideas to offer, and most importantly, they asked nothing for their time. They wanted nothing for themselves.

It was with this heritage in mind that the IOC mandated that the USOC be established under the guidance of volunteer leadership. Although this system worked well under the watchful eye of former President William Simon (1981-1985), today we are beginning to see inherent problems. The largest problem seems to be that a number of executives are in these positions for their self-fulfillment. Their personal agenda seems to have become more important than the movement.

For example, in my opinion, the Steinbrenner Overview Commission Report (which I will discuss later) was a farce, a worthless waste of time and money that didn't draw any real conclusions. But it did do a hell of a job convincing the media and the general public that George Steinbrenner was the right man to whip the old USOC back into shape.

Sadly, I feel the USOC is managed without vision, altruism, or determination today, though it certainly is not the way this organization should be managed. If the officers wish to run the day-to-day affairs, they should become day-to-day staff—and they should have the professional expertise to go with the various positions.

Another factor contributing to the organization's unrest and confusion is a certain parochial attitude by some individuals, much of which stems from the old factions in the debate between the AAU and the NCAA. Old foes don't seem to ever give up the battle; they just retreat, regroup, and once again attack.

If we look back at the reasons the Amateur Sports Act of 1978 was signed into effect, at the split between the NCAA and the AAU at that time, and at what has gradually happened to the leadership of the USOC since the Simon and Miller Show ended in 1985, we can see where the power resides. In 1978 the AAU leadership consisted, in part, of the men listed in the following box (one can also see where these gentlemen are today).

---

### WHERE THE PRE-AMATEUR SPORTS ACT
### AAU LEADERSHIP IS TODAY

| Official | 1978 position | 1990 position |
|----------|---------------|---------------|
| Bob Helmick | AAU President | USOC President |
| Ollan Cassell | AAU Executive Director | TAC Executive Director |
| Ray Essick | AAU Swimming Director | U.S. Swimming Director |
| Jim Fox | AAU Director Six Sports | USA Amateur Boxing Federation Director |
| Bill Wall | AAU Basketball Director | U.S. Amateur Basketball Director |

---

Who are the members of the USOC Executive Committee? What we really have is the same good-old-boy network that ran the AAU 12 years ago controlling the USOC today.

Again, I do not want to suggest that this is necessarily bad, but it wasn't the intent of the Amateur Sports Act to continue the old concept of elite federations responsible to the international federations running U.S. amateur sport. In my opinion, it is still important to have an independent authoritative board controlling amateur sport, particularly in this day and age where problems such as drug abuse transcend all sports.

It is also a problem that the USOC is controlled by the major sports. There are 41 Olympic sports, but track and field, basketball, swimming, boxing, hockey, gymnastics, figure skating, and wrestling have the majority of money, sponsor support, and television coverage. Some of these sports also benefit from the best developmental system for amateur sports in the country: the American collegiate system. If we look at the sports that the United States continues to excel in on the global level, we will find that the National Federation of State High School Associations (NFSHSA) and the NCAA, in particular, are still shouldering most of the load of training, developing, and preparing our young athletes for international competition.

The other sports take a minor role in the NCAA and other collegiate programs (such as those of the National Association of Intercollegiate Athletics and the National Junior College Athletic Association) and have very little opportunity to grow. The USOC should thus be the authority to provide equal opportunity to all the Olympic sports. Under the current leadership and policymakers, that is a doubtful outcome.

---

*Author's Note:*   By no means do I want the context of this argument to be mistaken as an endorsement for the NCAA. The NCAA is considered by many to be just as antiquated, just as mismanaged, as I feel the USOC has become, but that subject is for others to write about, not me.

---

Look at basketball, for example. Does anyone think the U.S. basketball team would be anywhere near as strong as it is today if it weren't for the NCAA program? Let's face it: Without March Madness there would be no Olympic gold, silver, or even bronze.

The same can be said about swimming. It is common knowledge among the athletes that if you can win a gold medal in the NCAA Swimming Championships, you'll have a great chance of winning an Olympic gold. One can travel the world and not find a more competitive meet (from top to bottom) than the NCAA's. The same can be said about track and field, and so on.

The sports that aren't part of the collegiate program, the sports that rely solely upon the USOC and their NGBs—such as team handball, ski jumping, luge, speed skating, bobsledding, weight lifting, and so on—are the ones in which we can't compete against the East Germans and Soviets. Why? Let's start with the USOC budget (see Figure 5).

The USOC operated with a budget of $149.9 million in the quadrennium of 1985 to 1988, its largest ever. Much of that money went to athlete assistance programs, such as the training centers and sports medicine programs, but how much of that money actually went directly to the athletes? 1.5 percent! That averages roughly $60 per month for every athlete on the Olympic Team. Actually, many athletes in minor sports didn't even achieve the average.

Let's face it: We're living in the real world; athletes need to eat and support themselves just like anyone else. We can argue this point forever, but in my mind, the days of true amateurism are long gone. In early days, an athlete might have been able to work as a banker, doctor, accountant, whatever, and still perform on the athletic field as a hobby.

These days, though, the performance has reached such a high level that this just isn't possible anymore. Someone who wants to be a great athlete has to devote himself or herself to the cause full time. There are no ifs, ands, or buts about it. Some athletes need to commit over 40 hours per

| Budget Item | Dollars Allocated (millions) | Percent of Budget |
|---|---|---|
| Operation Gold | 2.2 | 1.5 |
| Improvements | 4.7 | 3.1 |
| Olympics | 8.4 | 5.6 |
| Events/ competitions | 11.4 | 7.6 |
| Games planning | 12.1 | 8.1 |
| Sports medicine and science | 12.9 | 8.6 |
| Development grants | 16.7 | 11.1 |
| Miscellaneous | 18.1 | 12.1 |
| Training centers | 19.9 | 13.3 |
| Administration | 20.8 | 13.9 |
| Fund raising | 22.7 | 15.1 |
| Total | 149.9 | 100.0 |

**Figure 5.** USOC budget for the 1985-1988 quadrennium.

week to reach the physical conditioning and level of skill they need to succeed in their sport.

So the logical question becomes this: If an athlete is spending this much time on the practice field, how does she feed herself? Conversely, if she is working to keep her family afloat, how can she train enough to remain competitive? Often, I have found, that isn't very easy.

One should remember that in East Germany or the Soviet Union, athletes are taken care of by the state. Most are given a commission in their country's armed forces. This position takes care of their living and housing expenses, and so on.

For example, in Cuba the number of developing boxers in the state-supported system is 2,000. In East Germany before the 1988 Olympics, the number was 5,000. There are only about 200 developing American amateur boxers who ever see the Olympic Training Center or receive Sports Medicine and Science direct support. (I chose boxing as an example because amateur boxing is not a collegiate sport and must provide for its own development system.)

In the United States the athletes are usually on their own. So many are faced with the real-world decisions of having to find a means for survival. Unfortunately, this takes a lot away from our Olympic effort because an athlete *cannot* effectively train full time and work full time. Often, great athletes are turned away from sport in this country because there's no future in it. Most of them have to get a "real" job sooner or later. Ultimately, throwing a discus, speed skating, or swimming just doesn't fit into their plans anymore.

Let's look at the lives of two hypothetical athletes, Irina Athlete, who competed for the Soviet Union, and Irene Athlete, who competed for the United States.

Irina Athlete was a team handball player who lived in Moscow. Early in her life, one of Irina's physical education teachers noticed her particularly impressive strength and ability to play team handball. Irina was enrolled in a special school, where she was taught the usual curriculum but was also trained and instructed by several of the Soviet Union's finest team handball coaches.

---

*Author's Note:* Soviet sport coaches are not only former athletes in their sports but are graduates of a physical education curriculum far superior to that in the United States. The curriculum is four times as long and much more in-depth than the U.S. model.

---

Irina's parents didn't have to worry about paying for her education and coaching because the government picked up the bill. Later Irina was allowed to enroll in a university where she received her education and continued her training and technique work with her team handball coaches. Like her teammates, she was given a nice dormitory room, food, and a monthly allowance to spend at her leisure.

By this time, Irina had become a world-class athlete. She was given the rare opportunity to travel around the globe to compete in various competitions. Again, Irina's government sports federation paid for all of her expenses.

After Irina graduated from her university, she was given a job that paid well in the government. This was a mere formality: Though Irina was indeed required to undergo job training, she was still allowed to concentrate 90 percent of her attention on her team handball training. She was given a nice flat in Moscow, close to her training facility, her family, and the coaches and trainers who worked with her. Irina's salary let her afford her flat, furnish it, perhaps purchase a car, pay her grocery bills, buy household goods, and so on. Irina even got enough money to take her boyfriend to the ballet, sometimes travel a bit, and perhaps buy some luxury items. Basically, for a Soviet citizen, Irina had it made.

She competed for a spot on the Olympic Team and made it, beating her friend Natalia for the position. Natalia, however, remained a candidate for future Olympics, with nothing really lost: Both athletes had secure jobs, education, and so on.

Irina maintained her level of excellence. Indeed, she went on to win a gold medal in the Olympic Games. She became a national hero as well as a sports ambassador for the Soviet Union.

More important, later in her life, now that Irina has grown a bit too old to compete as effectively as she once had, her government still takes care of her. By this time, Irina wants to marry and start a family, but she keeps her steady job with good pay.

Perhaps Irina would decide she wanted to get back in the sport after some time. Because she's a trained team handball expert, Irina would be asked to join the sport federation as a coach. Again, the government would take care of her. She would be brought in to instruct the next budding group of team handball players. As you can see, the cycle would repeat itself with the next generation.

Irina had a special talent. Her government saw that and made it possible for her to use her talent and support herself.

That's not the case with Irene Athlete. Irene Athlete also played team handball. She had the same desire and talent that Irina Athlete had. She lived in Chicago.

When Irene was a girl, she was a standout athlete. She had a cousin who played team handball who taught her the game, and she picked it up rather quickly. When Irene got to high school, there wasn't any team handball organization to join. So, Irene's parents helped her find a team handball club, which practiced a half hour from their home. To help her conditioning, Irene ran alone every morning for about 3 miles. In the after-noon after school, Irene's parents had to drive her to practice. They'd drive a half hour—Irene would do her homework in the car—and then sit and wait for Irene's 2-hour practice to end. Then they'd drive her back home. They did this 5, maybe 6 days per week. Moreover, Irene's parents had to pay for the gas to get her to practice, the club fees to pay for her coach, the team's gym time, and any equipment Irene needed to wear. Irene's parents also had to pay for her plane ticket or bus fare when the team had to travel to play its matches. They sacrificed their money and time gladly, though, because Irene was an aspiring young athlete with talent and a dream of someday playing in the Olympic Games.

Later it was time for Irene to go to college. There isn't any team handball in college—no scholarships—so Irene had to find a job as a waitress to help pay her tuition. Irene had to work 25 hours each week on top of her studying, so she only had about 10 hours each week to devote to her training.

Somehow Irene became good enough to earn a spot on the United States Team Handball Team. Irene was then allowed to go out and train at the United States Olympic Training Center in Colorado Springs. Given her golden opportunity, Irene opted to drop out of college and go train with the team.

When Irene got out to Colorado she was given a room to live in—along with three other athletes. The room at the Training Center was smaller than her dorm room in college. She got meals at the Training Center cafeteria and an allowance from her sport federation of about $30 per month. If Irene wanted to visit her family, 1,000 miles away, make long distance phone calls, buy a car, travel in Colorado, or anything, she had to come up with that money on her own. The $30 allowance just didn't cut it, so she got a job at McDonald's to help pay her way. Again, this took away from her training time.

Because her sport federation didn't have much money, when the team wanted to travel to Holland to compete in an international event, Irene had to chip in for the additional cost. She had to ask friends and family for loans, and she had to spend her own modest paycheck.

Irene did make the Olympic Team. She beat out her friend Mary for the position. Mary had the same background and spent herself just as Irene did. But now she's a nobody: no money, no education, no job, and an ignominious future. Even though Irene made the team, the team didn't do so well; they didn't even make the medal round. After all, most of her teammates were spread as thin as Irene was. They weren't nearly as polished as Irina and her teammates because they hadn't trained together nearly as much as the Soviets had.

Irene's Olympic experience was over. She was an aging athlete now, ready to start a new chapter in her life, but she didn't have any college degree. She didn't have a job; her only real work experience had been waiting tables and working a cash register. Maybe she could be a coach; no, there's no real demand for Irene in the coaching business.

To make matters worse, Irene played out the last 2 years on a bum knee injury that turned out to require surgical reconstruction costing her over $15,000. The federation covered injuries only up to $2,000 (very often the case in most minor sports, where some don't have any injury coverage at all and most don't cover health problems; that is a disgrace, in my opinion). If Irina got hurt, on the other hand, she would never see a bill for surgery, hospital care, or rehabilitation.

So Irene is now on her own, folks. Maybe she will find a way to go back to school. Maybe she will be able to find a husband and start a family. No guarantees.

Like Irina, Irene finds herself a 25-year-old former Olympian. Unlike Irina, her future is uncertain. In effect, she's back where she started, only older. All Irene has left are some team sweatsuits, some good memories, and the image of a dream gone by.

Does anyone really wonder, then, why we aren't beating the Soviets in sports like team handball? Who in their right mind would make that kind of sacrifice? Believe me when I say some of our finest potential Olympians are turned away by this very scenario.

Admittedly, this is a particularly bleak example. Fortunately, that isn't how things work in all sports.

Let's look at basketball, for example. John Athlete is a basketball player from Massachusetts. He's able to play basketball at his high school, and he demonstrates his particular star quality to college recruiters.

Coach Steve Fisher picks up on this kid's talent and offers him a scholarship to play for the University of Michigan. For playing basketball with the Wolverines, John is given a nice dorm room, meals, and so on. When he has to go to Atlanta to play in the NCAA tournament, Michigan pays his way. If he breaks his leg, Michigan takes care of him. In theory, all John really has to worry about is getting good grades, earning his degree, and playing basketball.

---

*Author's Note:*   If the NCAA were smart, it too would do a better job of taking care of athletes, or at least allow the athletes to take care of themselves. I want to again emphasize that this example is here just for the sake of argument, not as an endorsement of outdated NCAA ideology.

---

There's no problem keeping John motivated. If he's a great player in college, he knows darn well that he'll be able to play professional ball. That means big bucks: We're talking millions. John would be in good financial standing for the rest of his life if he could earn a nice pro contract.

Even if he doesn't make the pros, John will have the opportunity to earn a degree from one of the finest universities in the country to fall back on. Whether or not he'll take advantage of this opportunity is in his hands, but in theory he'll have the tools to carve out a life for himself.

The Olympic Games are but a stepping stone in the overall picture here. The United States Olympic Basketball Team can only benefit from this highly successful system. The players know that making the Olympic Team will help their market value in the pros. So who wouldn't want to make the team and bring home a gold medal in the process?

Basketball has a great system, but who's shouldering the load here? The USOC? USA Basketball? Not hardly. The USOC is only able to cash in on the products the collegiate and high school athletic associations have provided for it.

When we look at the sports where the high school and collegiate systems do not have a big hand in the development of the athletes, we notice the USOC isn't enjoying nearly as much team success. Of course, some exceptions to this rule exist, figure skating, gymnastics, archery, and equestrian included. One other exception would be the sport of boxing. There are few significant college or high school boxing programs in this country, but the U.S. is still able to field strong teams for international events. In fact, in the 1976, 1984, and 1988 Olympic Games, the United States Boxing Team fared quite well.

So the USOC must be doing something correctly, right? Not necessarily.

Remember, there is a professional incentive that drives young boxers toward greatness. To be the world champion means riches and fame. For many, this picture is far more appetizing than the scene in which they are living. I am a strong supporter of amateur boxing because this sport can be a ticket to bigger and better things. For some young athletes, boxing can be a key to get out of the ghetto. Even for the 98 percent who never achieve national prominence, they learn self-defense, self-respect, and something about self-initiative and self-confidence.

Remember also that boxing isn't a very expensive sport in comparison to sports like ice hockey, figure skating, or skiing. Often a young kid in the inner city can pick up the sport of boxing at little or no cost at his neighborhood Boys' Club or gym. Here he is taught to box, and through programs such as state Golden Gloves competitions, he is given the opportunity to face opponents in the ring.

Unlike participants in a sport like team handball, these kids don't have to travel hours to find a team. Unlike hockey players, they don't have to come up with hundreds of dollars for equipment. They still have to find a way to eat, however.

Much of the United States' success in amateur boxing should be attributed to the U.S. armed forces. For example, Ray Mercer, who won a gold medal in the 1988 Olympic Games in the heavyweight (91-kg [200.5-lb]) class, was allowed to train, box, and represent his country in the Olympics while an enlisted soldier in the U.S. Army. The Army accepted the responsibility for training, housing, feeding, and paying

Mercer. I'm sure he'd tell you that was a key reason why he was able to win.

Once again, we can see that the USOC isn't necessarily shouldering the load of grooming and supporting young talent in all minor sports. Unfortunately, this lack of adequate support is hurting American performances at the Olympic Games. We need to direct more money away from USOC administrative overhead and toward the athletes in minor sports, particularly through training opportunities and services, if we want to keep them interested in competing in the Olympic Games and to give the interested ones the opportunity to devote their time to training. The Eastern Europeans do this.

This means the athletes need some guarantees—and I don't mean just putting money in their pockets and sending them off to train. We must spend more money on direct athlete care and development programs, entailing more centers available for full training, professional coaches, educational opportunities, health and injury insurance, disability coverage, nonsport career opportunities, and, most important, a life-after-sport opportunity program. This would be but a small payback to athletes who represent you and me and the good old U.S.A. in the international arena. Remember, the USOC doesn't go to the Olympics: The United States does, and the USOC has an obligation to ensure that the United States is well represented.

True amateurism probably isn't possible anymore. We need to stop shooting ourselves in the foot by clinging to an outdated ideal.

The program that dispersed 1.5 percent of the 1985-88 USOC budget (roughly $2.2 million) to the athletes was called Operation Gold. In addition to that, roughly $30 million was given to the various NGBs for athlete assistance. That averages out to about $200,000 per year for each NGB—far less than what's really needed. Furthermore, very little of that reached the athletes directly.

I should interject here that things have begun to change for the 1992 quadrennium. The USOC is making strides forward in terms of tuition assistance. The USOC is now offering up to $5,000 to certain athletes to defray costs of school. The USOC has an Olympic Job Opportunities Program (OJOP), which places athletes in work environments conducive to both career advancement and athletic achievement. In fact, the USOC was able to place 175 athletes in the OJOP before the 1988 Games. I think that's outstanding!

But the USOC has to expand these programs as soon as possible, because it still isn't doing enough. The USOC is headed in the right direction. My argument isn't that the USOC doesn't care: It's that the USOC could do more. These programs should be given priority number one status. The USOC could be much, much more thorough. It could offer athletes complete health benefits. It still has a long way to go before I'm convinced it is distributing funds to athletes with great effectiveness.

In fact, I still see examples of how the USOC is, in my opinion, poorly distributing funds. For example, in 1990 the USOC landed a $30-million TV deal. This revenue will be divided among the 41 NGBs. Each NGB will receive at least $100,000 in additional assistance, yet the major sports will receive the lion's share. I think this is a bit foolish because for the sports that really need the money, such as team handball, $100,000 won't do a whole lot of good. Thus, it only seems like the rich will get richer and the poor will stay about the same. I think the USOC has to realize where collegiate and high school programs are helping the Olympic effort, then target for more financial assistance the sports that aren't covered by such program overlaps. One would think the USOC should at least divide the $30 million evenly, that is, *if* all $30 million does find its way out of the USOC money pot to begin with.

Unfortunately, because revenues go through so many hands before they reach the athletes, many NGBs are virtually starved for funds. In fact, even major sports like boxing are sometimes left struggling to fill in the gaps when USOC support can't cut it. Interviewed for a brilliant 1988 *Sports Illustrated* article on the USOC titled "An Olympian Quagmire," USA/ABF Executive Director Jim Fox said, "We're top-heavy with our money. Only about 20 percent of the USOC's budget goes to the national governing bodies, which in terms of direct athlete support is where the rubber meets the road."[29]

Because the international federations, the IOC, and the USOC could each do a better job of filtering money to the athletes, the NGBs are often so strapped for funds that they have to go out and solicit corporate sponsors on their own, sometimes competing directly against the USOC for financial support.

So where did the money the USOC earned for the last quadrennium go? Well, over 40 percent of the USOC quadrennium budget is swallowed up by overhead: Staff, travel expenses, operations, and fund-raising activities alone accounted for over 40 million dollars. That's way too much.

In 1987 the USOC spent money to fly the House of Delegates to Washington, D.C., and put up over 300 people in hotel rooms for this meeting. I can't help but think this money could have been better spent on the eve of the Games. Fortunately, enough other people within the USOC felt the same way, and the USOC will avoid this expense from now on.

During the 1988 Olympic Winter Games in Calgary, USOC President Helmick ordered a study into USOC functions to see how it could become a more streamlined, productive governing body. While the study failed bitterly to suggest any innovative or imaginative ideas on what to do with more money, should the USOC receive it, it did divert attention from our team's dismal performance at Calgary. Moreover, the Overview Commission suggested that only "elite" athletes be targeted for assistance.

The USOC has set a target budget for the 1989-1992 Olympic quadrennium at $248 million. It expects to earn 40 percent of this budget through corporate sponsorships. Before the big corporation chiefs pull out their checkbooks for the USOC, though, I hope they will demand to know how and where their money will be spent.

Of that budget, the USOC hopes to give many of our Olympic athletes financial help from the USOC Athlete Assistance Program, a program designed to put more money in the pockets of U.S. athletes. Qualifying under various requirements, athletes will now be able to receive an extra few thousand dollars—and that should make some difference. In fact, the few athletes who meet USOC Athlete Assistance Program Level 2 Requirements, meaning they have dependents or extraordinarily high training costs, will receive a few thousand dollars more in additional direct financial assistance.

That's good, but most of this will go to our elite athletes in the highly visible, lucrative sports. Some of our track-and-field stars earn as much as $300,000 to $500,000 a year, and often $5,000 to $10,000 won't make much difference to them. On the other hand, it would make a big difference to aspiring junior-level athletes or athletes in "minor" sports.

Most Americans, including many USOC members, judge our Olympic success by an overall medal count. I think this is both ridiculous and dangerous. "Go for the gold!" "Gold fever!" "Bring home the gold!" I can't emphasize enough how narrow-minded this medal-hungry approach to sport is. In fact, it is this drive for gold medals, this belief that success can be measured only with a medal count, that has turned many young athletes on to drugs in the first place. The gold medal mentality is destroying the Olympic spirit in this country.

It would be nice if Americans would respect and admire an Olympic Team for more than the number of medals it can bring home. Yet, that is probably unrealistic. In 1992 many will hear or read that the Eastern Europeans won three times more medals than the United States did at the Olympic Games and then wonder how our team got so "bad."

The answer is obvious. The USOC focuses all its attention and resources into the major sports, whereas the Eastern Europeans develop *all* their Olympic programs. Often, the minor sports yield the most medals. For example, in 1984 there were 23 medals handed out in the various canoeing competitions. The U.S. took one. Twenty-four fencing medals were awarded. The U.S. took one.

Sure, the U.S. won in basketball, men's volleyball, and so on, but in each of these sports only three medals were awarded. So, for every medal the U.S. wins, the Soviets take three simply because they care about their minor sports programs.

The first point here is that it is stupid to gauge our Olympic success with a medal count because it isn't a fair reflection of American performances. The second point is that if the USOC wants to increase the overall percentage of medals American athletes win, it should stop overlooking sports like canoeing and fencing when it comes time to allot financial assistance. Most NGBs are still being deprived of well-deserved support. In short, the USOC has to spread the wealth more evenly and more effectively. The USOC still has a lot of overhead and administrative fat that needs to be trimmed.

There is one other aspect of our Olympic movement that needs to be reassessed: our Olympic Training Center project. We have two real Centers, in Colorado Springs and in Lake Placid, New York. There is also a small underutilized Center in Marquette, Michigan. Plans are also under way for a new Center to be built in San Diego.

The concept of having centralized multisport Olympic Training Centers is good in theory, but it hasn't worked out so well in the United States. One of the major problems with these Training Centers is that they're not easily accessible. To travel to any of these Centers can often be an all-day ordeal. Seventy percent of our track-and-field athletes live in California; who in their right mind would want to leave sunny Southern California to train in Colorado Springs? What hockey player would leave his hometown of Minneapolis to train in Lake Placid?

What's worse, our Training Centers are ill-equipped to adequately house and train athletes. The Colorado Springs Center doesn't even have an Olympic pool, it has only one gym, and the athlete housing would be graded subpar to most college dormitories. There's no throwing field. The track can be used only 6 months of the year. The list goes on. Is it any wonder why so few athletes choose to train here?

In Lake Placid the luge/bobsled run is literally decaying. The speed skating oval is usable only in very cold weather because, unlike with most modern facilities, the ice melts in moderate temperatures. We can't build a new oval because the chemical system used to cool the old one would be an environmental hazard if destroyed. Thus, most of our finest speed skaters ignore the facilities offered by the USOC and train in Milwaukee or Calgary. In fact, the great majority of American winter Olympians must train in Canada or Europe because the facilities available to them in their own country are terribly inadequate.

Clearly, in some respects the USOC lacks vision and forethought. I have no doubt that everyone involved wants to see the U.S. team be the best it can be. But with no method to this madness, that just isn't happening.

Track and field, swimming, and basketball, as examples, are successful for one reason: the high school and intercollegiate sports systems. Smaller sports could have the same opportunity if our high school and collegiate systems could financially support their development, but that is impossible. Often, when athletes who compete in these sports want to dip into the USOC money pot for training assistance, they find that it's empty.

That just shouldn't happen.

# 10

# Writing on the Wall

## My Final Days Inside the Five Rings

The early months of 1987 marked the beginning of my own end as the director of Sports Medicine and Science of the United States Olympic Committee.

At the Pan-American Games in 1987, a man I considered to be the most effective leader and spokesman the USOC has ever known, General George Miller, USAF, ret., "resigned" as the secretary general of the USOC. The previously untold reasons behind Miller's resignation were key indicators to me of just how mismanaged and political this business can be.

General Miller was a self-made man, and a former lieutenant general and vice commander of the United States Strategic Air Command. Quite honestly, Miller didn't need the USOC, at least not nearly as much as it needed him. He was in this business for one reason: He truly loved the athletes. Because he was an articulate speaker, a hard-charger, and a very thoughtful, logical person, he was the right man for the job. That wasn't only my opinion. A prominent search committee led by William Simon spent months before selecting him for his position over a great many applicants.

Unfortunately, today individuals like Gen. Miller are becoming harder and harder to find in the USOC, and Miller's fate was to get caught up in the ongoing battle of egos among the USOC officers and the Executive Committee.

Dick Abel, a former Air Force brigadier general and director of public affairs for the Secretary of the Air Force, was the director of the USOC's public relations division. General Abel was responsible for lobbying both the U.S. Congress and state legislatures to pass the important tax check-off or rebate legislation to benefit amateur sport. In this highly visible position, he received more attention than the officers and, ultimately, ran afoul of Helmick. In January 1987 Secretary General Miller was told to fire Abel, but Miller said he had no grounds to do so, and he dug his heels in for as long as he could.

Finally, in April 1987, after the USOC officers visited Korea on the premise that they would organize security measures for the team, only to find that Abel had already been there for that reason (and had thus preempted much of their need to be there), they forced Secretary General Miller to level the axe on Abel. Interestingly, no one was appointed to replace Abel in the position.

---

*Author's Note:*   A more recent example of this treatment is the ''resigna-tion'' of USOC Executive Director Baaron Pittenger, who was unaware that he was slated for retirement until he read the news in an executive memo.

---

Gen. Miller's problem was that he was almost too good. He was a dynamic individual. I had the acute sense that, from the very beginning, Helmick regarded Gen. Miller's very presence within the USOC as an indirect threat, and a power struggle seemed to be looming on the horizon. On the side of Helmick, from the very first day Gen. Miller was hired, were the NGB Executive Board members. They had never approved of Miller's hiring from Day 1. They wanted one of their own volunteer buddies to be moved to that position. It seemed inevitable to me that one way or another, this conflict was going to come to blows. There just didn't seem to be room in the enormous USOC bureaucracy for both Miller and Helmick.

Later in 1987 Douglas Roby, one of the two U.S. members on the IOC Executive Committee, resigned, leaving the opportunity for President Helmick to appoint himself to this position. Then, as fate would have it, Julian K. Roosevelt, the second American member of the Committee, died, leaving another opening on the IOC Executive Committee. Obvious candidates were Bill Simon, F. Don Miller, and of course George Miller. West German Horst Dassler, originator and owner of Adidas, was so impressed with Miller that he nominated him for the job. Helmick, however, didn't think it appropriate for a staff member, even one with Miller's credentials, to be the appointee. The NGB executives agreed, so Miller was blackballed. Support was thrown behind former athlete, and head of the Amateur Athletic Foundation of Los Angeles, Anita DeFrantz. She was certainly an excellent choice, but the politics involved were interesting nonetheless.

I subsequently learned that a certain NGB executive informed Dassler that Miller would not be a good choice because he was going to be "gotten rid of" in the near future. This was another nail in Miller's coffin and the beginning of his (and my own) end with the USOC. The innuendo was that George Miller had overstepped his bounds as a staff person and that this type of action would not be tolerated. The word was clearly out: Get rid of Miller. Helmick actually tried to have Miller fired at the 1987 Executive Committee meeting in Reno, Nevada, but cooler heads among the officers prevailed.

Then came the events of the 1987 Pan-American Games in Indianapolis. USOC protocol requires the day-to-day staff to assume a low profile and take a backseat to the officers when international events roll around. Unfortunately, important incidents take place in these events that require expertise—and expertise in sport diplomacy is something I believe many officers lack. This problem surfaced several times at the 1987 Pan-American Games.

The first incident of this type involved a Chilean shooter who was denied a U.S. visa by Assistant Secretary of State Elliott Abrams. The reason? The Chilean was a known member of a Chilean right-wing hit squad. He was reported to be an assassin, thus certainly, in my mind, an outrageous example of an amateur athlete. Helmick, however, disapproved of Abrams's action, hinting that the government should stay out of such sports-related issues, and that infuriated the State Department.

Someone had to answer repercussions from the State Department on behalf of the USOC, and because Helmick left Indianapolis to return to his law practice in Des Moines, Gen. Miller did. Miller's reaction was that the State Department was correct: Although any athlete is entitled to represent his country if appointed, countries should have the responsibility to not allow suspected criminals to be selected for their national teams. Thus, the State Department won out.

This little public differing of opinions didn't sit well with the parties involved. This problem grew more volatile when Chilean fans and athletes, along with the Cubans, became rather restless. People began to fear that these countries would disturb the Games or lead a boycott. In fact, the Cuban team threatened to pull out of the Games and leave.

George Miller, in a publicized and highly complimented move, interceded, convincing Chile and Cuba to stay by inviting the president of the Havana Organizing Committee, Cuban Minister of Sport Hernandez, to come and accept the flag at the closing ceremonies on behalf of Havana, the 1981 host city—not a bad move to quell the unrest. Minister Hernandez, by the way, was the highest ranking Cuban official to visit the United

States in 25 years, and he was certainly the most powerful Cuban representative to participate—more visible than the type of official who might normally accept the flag in such circumstances.

It was also during this period that Bill Green, a U.S. hammer-thrower, was found positive for using banned anabolic-androgenic steroids. At that time, I first became aware of Bob Helmick's reluctance to involve himself in the drug issue. During a hearing between the officers and Bill Green (which included George Miller and me), Vice President Steve Sobel seemed to be the only one speaking. Most of his discussion was directed toward what the officers could do to get Green off the hook. As frustrations started to build, Green's coach suddenly shouted out, "What's wrong with you [USOC]? Are you more interested in getting rid of drugs than winning medals?"

George Miller, the only one with guts enough to stand up to the issue at hand, shouted back, "You got that right! Meeting adjourned."

Obviously, no further reasoning could have gone on, and I don't think the officers were very pleased. I was pleased—pleased with George Miller. Either we support a drug-free competition or we don't. In this case, it isn't "whatever it takes to win."

The final nail in Miller's coffin came when the Indianapolis organizing committee planned a most lavish party for the administrators of the Pan-American Sports Organization and requested a $100,000 USOC contribution to fund the budget override. President Helmick committed to it. George Miller, although responsible for the budget, had not been consulted. He thought sinking $100,000 into a party was improper, knowing that there wasn't money in the budget for this type of food, drink, and entertainment for nonathletes. After George Miller and the USOC treasurer, Howard C. Miller, challenged Helmick's decision, the USOC finally settled on allowing $50,000 to be spent on the party.

A few days later, on a Sunday morning at 8 a.m., Helmick, with Executive Committee approval, handed George Miller a prepared letter of resignation; Miller could either sign it or be fired by 2 p.m. In a subsequent personal conversation with me, George Miller chose the honorable way out rather than cause a big stir right in the heart of the premier amateur athletic competition of 1987. George's final comment to me was, "The only amateurs left in the Olympic movement are the officers and administrators."

When Gen. Miller resigned, I began to understand fully the lunacy that often controls the decision-making process in the USOC. This event sent a very powerful, negative message to me. It told me two things. First, the USOC volunteer executives were all-powerful. When push came to shove, it really didn't matter what the Olympic House staff said or did. Helmick was the main man. He called the shots. Period.

Second, I learned from Helmick's handling of Gen. Miller that to survive in the USOC, you have to be a yes-man, something I had never been before. It became clear to me at this point that sooner or later Helmick was going to be upset with something I said or did and that it would be only a matter of time before I was swept out of his way like Gen. Miller had been.

Understanding that Helmick was the only person with significant influence in this organization, and given what I had seen to be weak support of the drug issue, I knew if ever I stumbled in my highly visible drug-control position, it would be fatal. I was taken aback by the thought that, due to the sensitivity of the doping issue in sport, Helmick and the organization might not be there when times got tough with drug cases.

In the fall of 1987, the Canadian minister of sport invited George Walker (the executive director of the Council of Europe, an organization of Western European nations), the Canadian Olympic Committee, and the USOC to meet and discuss what could be done to stop drug abuse in sport. New Executive Director Baaron Pittenger agreed that the USOC should be involved with this process and appointed Don Catlin, MD—director of UCLA's Paul Ziffren Olympic Drug Testing Laboratory and chairman of the USOC Substance Abuse, Research, and Education Committee—and me to attend. Helmick attended but deferred to Catlin and me as the experts and decision makers. However, we were cautioned not to commit to any funding support. The meeting was very symbiotic, and we agreed to meet later in Paris to plan the blueprint for organizing the first World Conference on Doping in Sport.

The conference was held in Ottawa, Canada, in May 1988. Representatives from twenty-six countries attended, including East Germany and the Soviet Union. The delegates met for 3 days. The mission was to approve a worldwide antidoping charter agreement. Furthermore, we were to carry the document resulting from this conference to the IOC Executive Committee and President Juan Antonio Samaranch at the 1988 Olympic Summer Games in Seoul.

The USOC was represented in Ottawa by President Helmick, Don Catlin, and me. Helmick stayed for the opening session and then left. Nonetheless, Catlin and I stayed. After 3 days of working, we helped the conference achieve a unanimously approved charter agreement, which was subsequently accepted by the IOC Executive Committee. More significant at the time was the germination of a USSR-USOC drug testing agreement.

The conference in Ottawa was set up in a United Nations type of format, with all the delegations from the various countries meeting in a giant theaterlike environment. Because the United States followed the Union of Soviet Socialist Republics in alphabetical order, we were seated just behind the Soviet delegation. Thus, Dr. Catlin and I had a golden opportunity to informally confer one-on-one with the Soviets regarding the doping problem in sport. After several discussions, we proposed to them for the first time the possibility of a bilateral antidoping agreement.

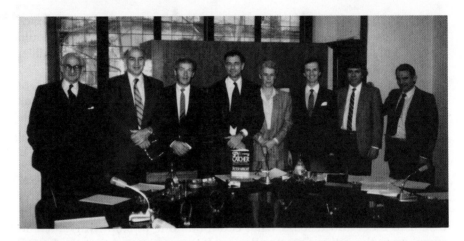

Participants at the May 1988 meeting in Paris, France, to plan the first World Conference on Antidoping in Sport held June 26-29, 1988, in Ottawa, Canada. From left to right: Sir Arthur Gold, representative from the United Kingdom; Don Catlin; Bob Voy; Prince Alexandre de Merode, Chairman of the IOC Medical Commission; Abby Hoffman, Director of Sport from Canada; Lyle Makosky, Assistant Deputy Minister of Fitness and Amateur Sport in Canada; Robert Dugal, Director of the IOC drug lab in Montreal and an IOC Medical Commission member; and George Walker, head of the Council of Europe Sport Section from Strasbourg, France.

A dual nation testing policy: We test you guys, you test us—that sort of thing. Oddly enough, the Soviets were interested.

Upon our return to the United States, Pittenger and Helmick were informed, and they agreed to allow Dr. Catlin and me to set up a meeting with the Soviets in Seoul during the Summer Games. But something very profound happened to me between this conference in Ottawa and the actual Olympic Games. It signalled for me that the handwriting was on the wall.

I've already mentioned the incident at the TAC Olympic Trials where eight tests turned up positive. All those tests were eventually appealed and won on the basis of accidental or inadvertent use.

That's not all there was to the story, though. Just prior to the Olympic Games, USOC Media Relations Director Mike Moran conducted an open house in Colorado Springs for approximately 100 journalists from across the nation. He asked if I would give a 2-hour presentation. Having given presentations to the journalists many times over the prior 4 years, I knew them well, and I understood they would expect the same openness they had grown to appreciate from me in the past. I was supposed to give them both barrels, with slides and so on—the whole show.

And I did. I felt it was an excellent opportunity to tout some of the successes of our drug testing and allay a lot of old rumors. I had done this type of thing hundreds of times before, and, quite honestly, the media always responded well and gave the USOC a pat on the back. So I talked about pre-Games preparations, the living conditions in Seoul, and what exactly the USOC Sports Medicine Department was doing to help the athletes get ready for the Games.

In addition, I made public the aggregate number of positive drug tests over the last 5 years. This was important to prove that the drug testing process was on the right track.

Well, as I should have anticipated, I was asked, "Were there any positive tests at the TAC trials?"

I thought that was a good question, a fair question. It needed an honest answer, even though final appeals had not yet been heard and we weren't sure that the positive tests represented doping. Besides, no one would believe *nothing* was found at the trials.

So I told the person who asked this question, "Yes, there were eight positive tests at this event. The athletes in question were positive, and the appeal process—to determine if it was truly doping or whatever—is in the works."

That seemed to be a fair, honest answer. I didn't criticize anyone. I didn't name names. I told the truth.

What was I going to do, lose my hard-earned respect from the media and say there were no positives? They would have eventually heard differently from USOC and TAC officialdom. Besides, if you tell the truth, you can't get in trouble, right?

Wrong. When I let the cat out of the bag that there were eight positives at the TAC trials, I earned a permanent membership on the USOC Executive Committee's and TAC's shit lists.

In fact, when word filtered back to the Olympic Committee that I had answered this question, the initial response was, "Dr. Voy should learn to keep his f---ing mouth shut."

Not "He's right" or "He's telling the truth" but "Dr. Voy should learn to keep his f---ing mouth shut."

That really upset me. If the people want to know the answer to a question, if they want to know what's going on with the selection of their Olympic Team, I feel like I ought to give them an honest answer. Others, I guess, do not.

All the problems with subsequent misunderstandings, both at home and abroad, that the USOC was suppressing test results would have easily been avoided if both Helmick and USOC Executive Director Pittenger had promptly supported my statement and explained the possibility that this represented innocent use. Instead, the Administrative Committee instructed

Pittenger to muzzle me. I was no longer permitted to speak on the issue, which only made the USOC look like they were covering something up. Therefore, I entered the Olympic Games unable to say anything about drugs, testing—anything—from that point on because I thought if I did say anything, I'd lose my job. I wasn't allowed to answer the questions I had been answering for the USOC for the previous 4 years anymore.

Remember that at that time the organization was going through an anabolic-androgenic steroid appeal with swimmer Angel Myers. We were also hearing appeals by various boxers who had tested positive for drugs at the box-offs.

But I was muzzled. So, when the Olympics in Seoul finally rolled around, my sole responsibility was to be an assistant to Baaron Pittenger and not be involved in the drug control program of the Games. This was a difficult position to be in, particularly considering the fact that I had been given a position with the IOC Medical Commission in charge of testing at the Games. It also harmed my credibility with the Soviets on the USOC/USSR testing agreement. I was simply a private advisor to Pittenger in case the drug question came up again.

And did the drug question come up again! I remember the night I first heard that Ben Johnson had tested positive for anabolic-androgenic steroids. I was awakened in the middle of the night by a secretary from NBC. She wanted to know if I would be willing to appear on "NBC Nightly News" with Tom Brokaw to speak about the drug situation. I said I would, but, knowing that I was not permitted to speak for the USOC on the issue, I suggested that she seek President Helmick's permission. She then asked if she could call Helmick for me, because I had just been awakened and it was necessary for me to appear within 2 hours. I agreed; she made the call.

This evidently embarrassed Helmick. In addition to chastising me for telling NBC that I needed his permission to speak, he insisted on meeting with me to rehearse what I was to say. I had been trusted by the USOC to speak on television unrehearsed for 4 years, but now I had to appear before Helmick and a volunteer PR person. As nervous as I was in anticipating appearing live on national television on such a significant issue, I thought the plan of rehearsing was unnecessary, especially when only a 10- to 15-second response would be required.

Eventually, after being asked several hypothetical questions, I told Helmick that I thought this was ridiculous. His response: "I don't want to get in a pissing match with you." And he left. This wasn't an endearing comment and vote of confidence for someone about to speak for the USOC. As I predicted, however, the interview amounted to no more than a couple of statements that, in my opinion, went very well.

Nonetheless, that little episode convinced me that my days were numbered, and I was correct. After having helped lay the groundwork for the USSR-USOC drug testing agreement and having just met with the Soviet delegation in the village, I was informed that I was no longer a member of the committee working on this agreement. That was a blow. I then knew, based on how I had seen the system work before, that being a marked staff member meant I would be gradually relieved of responsibility and excluded from the progressive programs.

My being ignored and excluded became more evident as time wore on. Yet, I stayed on through the winter of 1988-89 because word was out that the Sports Medicine and Science Department was being critically looked at by the Administrative Committee and that its future in the next quadrennium was at stake. Not only the science program but also the education program and library resources were being slated for extinction. Therefore, I had much more to accomplish: to save the programs I felt were so valuable to the athletes. Rather than leave after the Games, I decided to take my chances with the powers that be and fight for what was important overall.

One might remember, earlier that year the United States sent its winter Olympic Team to compete in the 1988 Olympic Winter Games in Calgary, Canada, and the team did poorly, bringing home only two gold medals. Shaken, perhaps, by our less-than-satisfying showing, and anxious to divert public attention, President Helmick called on USOC Vice President George Steinbrenner III to conduct an internal investigation of the USOC to see how we could streamline our Olympic effort. Steinbrenner was to pinpoint the areas where the USOC let the team down. I had no problem with that: seemed like a good idea, a much needed reassessment of our operation as a whole. However, all of the commission's members came from the Executive Board. Once again, the fox was guarding the henhouse.

I did have a problem with the fact that Helmick ordered the study to take place right in the middle of the Olympics. I thought that was a tremendous vote of no confidence to the athletes who had yet to compete in the Games. Nevertheless, I thought Olympic House and the Center for Sports Medicine and Science would now be given the opportunity to offer our insights—including some direct feedback from the athletes—on the problems facing the U.S. Olympic movement.

Unfortunately, I was wrong. I asked Executive Director Baaron Pittenger when I would be allowed to interview with the Steinbrenner Commission. Pittenger informed me that the Commission would probably not even come to the Center for a discussion. He further stated that he was the only staff member scheduled to report to the commission. He would, of course, speak for the Division of Sports Medicine and Science.

Now, I had (and still have) a great amount of respect for Baaron Pittenger, but it made no sense that he should be the one to represent Sports Medicine and Science at this interview. The President of the United States does not report on the activities and problems of the Defense Department before a Congressional hearing; why should Pittenger be the one to field all the questions we had hoped to answer? In fact, my staff and I had spent days brainstorming the issues and had come up with our recommendations for the future as well as the wish list for Sports Medicine and Science in the 1990s. In addition, the upcoming USSR-USOC drug testing agreement and the growing monster of drugs in sport demanded new ideas and a budget commensurate to meet future needs.

Someone with more direct experience certainly could have been helpful to the Commission, but the Commission did not see fit to ask any of the experts how we thought the drug problem was threatening the Olympic ideal or how we should approach eliminating this problem. Thus, the Steinbrenner report was compiled with no direct input from the Sports Medicine and Science Department or, to my knowledge, the Olympic Training Center staff.

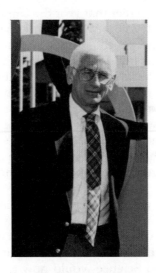

Baaron Pittenger

When it finally came out in early 1989, the Steinbrenner report was all that I expected: not worth the money spent on it. All the issues raised were well known to the staff and could have been compiled from the minutes of a handful of George Miller's weekly staff meetings. But then the members of the Commission probably spent most of their time learning what the USOC operation was really all about to begin with. What a wasted opportunity to get real direction! My opinion of the Commission is that it was constituted simply to deflect negative public opinion. Period.

The final straw to break my effort to remain effective for the USOC was the 1989-92 budget deliberations. The USOC was increasing its proposed budget for the next quadrennium by nearly $100 million; the 1985-88 budget had been $149.9 million. The new budget: $248 million. Traditionally, Sports Medicine and Science had received about 10 to 11 percent of the overall USOC budget each quadrennium since its inception. After diligent brainstorming and creation of a vision statement for the nineties, we in Sports Medicine and Science proposed a $36-million budget.

Admittedly, it was a dream budget. But it was also a creative plan that not only met the expected needs of the direct athlete services—that is, clinics, insurance, and so on—but it also increased monies available for research and development. More important, our plan called for a functional change in priorities that would allow more money for each of 39 NGBs to establish their own sports medicine and science services (there were only 39 Olympic sports at that time). This all represented a modest increase, from 10 or 11 percent, to 15 percent of the overall USOC budget.

We understood well that the plan probably wouldn't fly on its own, but, as with any other business proposal, we opted to shoot for the moon. Though we knew we might land a little short, we hoped we could get a lot more than originally expected.

The first budget go-around made it apparent that we were out of our minds. After considerable dickering, we submitted our absolute bottom figure, which would allow only a modest increase but, at the least, a maintenance of services and a provision for some expansion: $18.2 million. This number was then arbitrarily, without counsel or explanation, slashed by the Executive Committee by $5 million, putting us back to the 1985-88 quadrennial running budget of $13.2 million, or a reduction of overall raise from the traditional 10 or 11 percent to 7.3 percent. My staff members and I were later able to salvage some of the $5 million: $1 million was restored to the plan but earmarked only for the USSR-USOC drug testing agreement.

What did all this mean to Sports Medicine and Science?

- Continuation only of the program of physiologic and biomechanic testing of NGB athletes, and of only the few who visited the Colorado Springs Olympic Training Center
- No expansion of the valued national toll-free drug control hotline used by athletes, coaches, and educators
- *No* sports science *research*

Because I pleaded that the only part of the USOC to suffer from this would be the athletes, and later the sports officials themselves, it was apparent from Administrative Committee attitudes that this was a vote of no confidence for my program. The USOC will argue that the overall percentages of other divisions were also cut. However, these divisions, unlike Sports Medicine and Science, had more actual money allocated for the new quadrennium. For example, the fund-raising budget percentage decreased from 15.5 percent to 11.5 percent, but the dollar amount allocated was increased from $22 to $26 million.

What this budget fiasco did was strip our athletes of some of the services we had been able to offer them before 1988—this at a time when all attention suggested that our Olympic failures were caused by not providing the athletes with *enough* resources. How were they affected? The following box shows how the cuts snuffed out Sports Medicine and Science.

## EFFECTS OF BUDGET CUTS
## ON SPORTS MEDICINE AND SCIENCE

| Program | Amount of cut (percentage) |
| --- | --- |
| General administrative operations | 22 |
| Drug testing | 33 |
| Exercise-induced bronchospasm study | 100 |
| Nutrition education and counseling | 74 |
| Sport science (physiology, biomechanics, sport psychology, computer and engineering services) | 25 |
| Coaches' education | 60 |
| Sports Medicine and Science research grants | 80 |
| Education and library services | 15 |

In my final months at the USOC, I couldn't believe what I was seeing and hearing. The USOC planned to raise $100 million more dollars, and not a penny of it was to go to Sports Medicine and Science. The Executive Committee was trying to tell me something. My effectiveness had not only been decreased, but it was obvious to me that it was not deemed valuable.

I resigned my position March 17, 1989, after 5 years and 3 months of service. In many ways it had been fun, but it was time to move on. I hoped there would be other ways to contribute to sport in the future. I felt that if I was truly to help the athletes and do whatever it took to clean up sport, I would have to find other routes and formulate new solutions for our problems.

So I have.

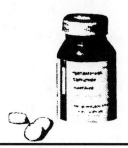

# Prescription
# for Reform

# 11

## A Level Field
## of Play

### How Doping Control
### Could Work

Where do we go from here? How *can* we rid amateur sports of drugs?

Let me start by saying this is a fight we'll all have to join if it will ever be won.

Sport administrators have to decide they want drugs out of sports, and they have to back their words with action.

Athletes have to decide they don't want to compete on an uneven playing field. They have to pressure for action and commitments. They have to learn to recognize empty promises when they hear them.

Coaches have to teach kids that being the best they can be doesn't necessarily mean doing whatever it takes to win. They have to be aware of the drug problem and, above all, be concerned with the welfare and health of their athletes.

Corporate sponsors who fund the whole amateur sports business have to demand fairness for all athletes—*before* they write the big checks. As successful businessmen, corporate leaders should at least want to be aware of what they're investing in.

Parents have to be sensitive to the drug problem. It isn't always the neighbor's kid who runs into trouble. A little more support and a little less pressure at home could go a long way.

People have to stop placing the biggest, strongest, and most abrasive athletes on pedestals for young kids to admire and respect. What ever happened to choosing role models who were not only great athletes but also class acts? I got sick of reading about Brian Bosworth in the mid- to late 1980s. Why did he deserve such attention? It wasn't because he was that great a player; his career in the pros can attest to that. It was because he was a wild man, and the American public ate it up.

I know I can't fault the media for covering the stories the general public wants to buy. But consider this. In early 1989 *Sports Illustrated* ran a story about Benji Ramirez, the high school athlete from Ashtabula, Ohio, who died of a heart attack while on anabolic-androgenic steroids. This excellent story had impact, to say the least. It clearly described the dangers of anabolic-androgenic steroid use, and it outlined how Ramirez was led down his fatal path of AAS use by an insatiable desire to be "big." He couldn't have enough muscles. Muscles were power, and power was happiness. All he cared about was pumping up, and it ultimately killed him.

Just weeks after this tear-jerking story was run, *Sports Illustrated* featured former Michigan State University lineman Tony Mandarich on its cover. Inside, a story painted a portrait of a caffeine-guzzling, iron-pumping muscle maniac who may or may not have been on steroids (we were supposed to draw our own conclusions; I've drawn mine). It just seems odd to me: Tony Mandarich is the type of guy Benji Ramirez probably would have idolized.

Average, run-of-the-mill fans have to scrutinize sports and sports heroes more carefully. After all, they are the reason for the show to go on.

Everyone has to get involved, because all the doctors in the world won't make much of an impact until an overriding atmosphere of commitment and concern surfaces in sport. I can only offer some ideas that I have developed throughout my years working both inside and outside the five rings and invite others to conjure up some of their own. Unfortunately, there doesn't seem to be one clearcut blueprint to solving the problems that face us today. There are certainly steps that can and should be taken, however.

The problems with performance enhancing drugs: (a) they work; (b) athletes can use some drugs in a way that allows them to slip through the current dope testing system; (c) athletes believe if they don't use drugs they will be at a disadvantage competing; and (d) many types of drugs are *not* illegal to use.

Though selling anabolic-androgenic steroids without a medical prescription is a punishable crime, possession and personal use of these substances is not. Also, it certainly isn't illegal to get hold of anabolic-androgenic steroids with a doctor's prescription. Unfortunately, many physicians are willing to prescribe these drugs to athletes with little understanding of the dangers they pose. If doctors do not feel ethically compelled to stay out of the anabolic-androgenic steroid business with the athletes, maybe we should legally compel them to do so with tough laws prohibiting such unethical practices and dishing out severe penalties for those who break these laws.

In addition, many athletes feel so long as they're not breaking any law by using these drugs, they aren't really doing anything wrong. I can't tell you how many athletes have said, "Why shouldn't I use steroids? If they're not in my system when I'm competing and if it isn't against the law to use them, what's the big deal?"

The big deal, as I've explained, is that these drugs can give the user an unfair advantage over the competition by helping build muscle mass during training. Using anabolic-androgenic steroids is cheating.

Aside from their impact on sport, these drugs are wrong because they could potentially kill the user or cause serious long-term side effects. We just don't yet know the complete extent of the damage these drugs can cause. The athletes don't either, but they may learn the hard way.

Perhaps the biggest problems these drugs cause can be attributed to the impact AAS can have on the minds of users. Plain and simple, roid rage, the uncontrollable aggressiveness that may result from AAS use, can kill and injure. Remember the stories I told about the murders committed by people using AAS who literally couldn't control their aggression?

Anabolic-androgenic steroids can be just as volatile, just as addictive, and just as potent and deadly as cocaine, heroin, or any other controlled substance. In my mind, solution Number 1 is to treat these drugs accordingly.

## LAY DOWN THE LAW

Some states have already moved to classify anabolic-androgenic steroids under Category II of the Controlled Substances Act of 1970. That means if a person uses or possesses these drugs in those states without a bona fide prescription from a licensed physician, they're breaking the law just like if they were to use any other Category II drug, such as cocaine, heroin, or marijuana. Someone using anabolic-androgenic steroids or growth hormone would not only be a cheater but also a criminal. Someone caught with these drugs would be in trouble with the law. Period.

I think, after seeing firsthand how these drugs have ruined families and claimed lives, we have a very salient argument for placing all of these drugs on the list of Category II controlled substances nationwide. Such a move would probably help eliminate the drug problem among athletes. Also, when these drugs are rigidly controlled and classified under the same psychiatric definition as mind-influencing and addicting substances, then drug testing as well as detoxification and rehabilitation might be covered by health insurance. This would also allow sports medicine physicians a better opportunity to rehabilitate athlete addicts.

I hope people will check with their congressmen or senators to see how they feel about this issue and to ask these representatives to support tougher, all-inclusive antidrug legislation.

## IMPROVE RESEARCH

Another obvious step that I feel must be taken, if the problem of drugs in sport will ever be resolved, has to do with the amount of research done on this topic. There simply haven't been enough financial or human resources invested to help researchers and physicians combat the problem with much effectiveness. As I've said, some of this has to do with researchers' inabilities to conduct effective double-blind crossover studies, but there are other options to explore.

Remember, I discussed how part of the reason sport officials and the medical profession in general have had trouble convincing some athletes not to use drugs has to do with our lack of thorough knowledge on this subject. Believe me when I say that in some cases, a few real smart athletes who have been around the block a few times know more about anabolic-androgenic steroids, growth hormone, stimulants, beta-blockers, and so on than most doctors. There's much research data that can be acquired just by communicating with this group of athletes.

The drug abuse situation is most frightening when one considers the fact that many other athletes don't know *anything* about the drugs they're taking. They are told by their peers or their drug gurus that the drugs are safe and, if used as instructed, they don't have to worry. Besides, as we have seen, many athletes are willing to do whatever it takes to win, even if it means risking death. Most of the athletes I know to be using anabolic-androgenic steroids, whether they are willing to admit this or not, really aren't in a position to make an accurate judgment about the drugs they're taking. Many gurus aren't either.

Clearly, more resources must be directed toward the study of performance enhancing drugs and the roles these substances play in sport today. Let's get the facts laid out on the table in plain sight for everyone to see.

Unfortunately, even today, as the sports media continues to remind everyone of the impending doom these drugs spell for the sports world, very little has been done to help the nation's leading researchers provide us with answers. One of the leading experts on anabolic-androgenic steroids in the United States, Charles E. Yesalis, MPH, ScD, of Penn State University, explained this particular situation to me as follows:

> For the last half century experts in this field have consistently stated that the long-term effects of anabolic steroids are unknown. There are probably over one million anabolic steroid

users in the U.S. alone, most of whom lack the opportunity to make an informed judgement regarding their steroid use. On the other hand, individuals who consider cocaine, tobacco or alcohol use have had much more information available to them. Unfortunately, many current or potential anabolic steroid users mistake ''absence of evidence'' for ''evidence of absence.'' Even more frustrating is the fact that in two recent national studies, a majority of anabolic steroid users surveyed expressed intentions of stopping use if deleterious health effects were unequivocally established. Clearly, the lack of scientific information has impeded, if not precluded, the formulation of an effective health education strategy.

During the past five years our research team has approached the federal government on three occasions to fund a study of the long-term health effects of anabolic steroids. On each occasion we have been unsuccessful.

It is not an exaggeration to state that virtually all of the information on anabolic steroid abuse has been obtained without the support of the government or sport federations. Given that a significant number of *basic* questions on steroid abuse as it relates to health effects, levels of use and intervention strategies remain unanswered, the federal government as well as the NCAA and IOC need to accept the responsibility of funding research in this area.

If the federal government is serious about its War on Drugs, I see no reason why anabolic-androgenic steroids, growth hormone, and other performance enhancing substances shouldn't be included in the overall research and education program.

I, like Professor Yesalis, believe the NCAA, USOC, and IOC should get involved more with drug research. You can sit around and cry about the problem of drugs in sport for years, but that won't accomplish anything, particularly if no one involved has an adequate understanding of the beast they're dealing with. You can also invent all types of ''aggressive'' or ''progressive'' drug testing programs, but they too will realize only limited success if you really can't be sure of *what* you're looking for, *who* is using it, and *how* these drugs are being used.

For example, I recently read how the IOC has invested millions of dollars in its fight against drugs by creating a ''flying drug lab.'' The idea is to put a sophisticated drug testing facility in an airplane that could conceivably swoop down on athletic competitions around the world with little or no warning to the athletes.

Just how well will this idea ''fly''? Let's think about it. The really ''developed'' countries—countries where we find drug use most prevalent

—already have IOC-approved testing labs. Thus, such a flying lab would have little or no impact except in third-world "national" competitions. Also, when you consider how word of testing leaks in the athletic community, I seriously doubt that the IOC flying lab would have much effect on elite competitors whatsoever. When the big competitions roll around, the athletes are already well prepared to beat the tests. Thus, it wouldn't matter if you brought the lab in on a truck, bus, train, boat, or, yes, even a plane.

---

*Author's Note:*  The IOC has thrown support behind a flying lab, yet to date only a handful of IOC-approved labs exist. In the whole U.S., there are two. That's foolish: This type of lab technology should be freely exchanged among all interested universities, colleges, and science and research centers with a need and an interest, and drug labs should not be monopolized.

---

Aren't the people who came up with this flying lab idea really putting the cart before the horse? Considering its hefty price tag, I think it makes more sense to spend the money on increasing our overall research effort rather than on jet fuel. When we consider the enormous amounts of money the USOC and the IOC earn from television contracts and international corporate sponsorships, wouldn't it make sense to spend some of that money on drug research, education, and athlete rehabilitation? Unfortunately, many sport administrators would rather spend millions of dollars inventing all sorts of aggressive testing procedures. Many of the same people, such as the USOC Executive Board, have balked at the notion of research and education funding. That's just penny-wise and pound-foolish.

If sport federations are unwilling to shoulder this load, maybe corporate America could point the way. Perhaps one of the leaders in the pharmaceutical industry would like to begin a public relations program whereby it would establish itself as the lead sponsor of performance enhancing drug research, and drug testing for sports worldwide, becoming the guardian of fair play in Olympic sport, or the "official sponsor of fair play in Olympic sport."

Clearly *somebody* has to take the lead on this front. So long as corporate America keeps writing checks for the USOC, wouldn't it, too, have a stake in whether amateur sports can become drug free?

The main responsibility of the USOC is to serve the athletes. With athletes playing around with potentially lethal drugs, one of the best ways Sports Medicine and Science could help the USOC serve them is to offer some real knowledge on the drugs used in sport today—knowledge attainable only through research.

# INCREASE EDUCATIONAL EFFORTS

A step we should take to eliminate the problem of drug abuse among athletes is to increase our educational effort. I have always been a strong proponent for education as a means against doping in sport. As the medical research community learns more about performance enhancing drugs, we should make a strong effort to relay this information to young athletes across the country as quickly as possible.

This can be done many ways. The USOC already produces a number of brochures for athletes. There is also a national toll-free drug hotline number for athletes interested in knowing more on this subject; the USOC should make expansion of the hotline program one of its highest priorities.

More emphasis should be placed on educating younger athletes rather than those competing at the elite level. Remember, many drug-using athletes are first introduced to these drugs very early in life, some before they even reach high school. Many events, such as the United States Swimming Junior Nationals or the AAU National Junior Olympics, could include drug brochures in the "goodie bags" given to competitors at registration. I also think drug testing at this level is a must. That's where trouble starts; by the time athletes reach college, they are addicted and education is much less effective.

The government's antidrug educational campaign is being effectively spread into the nation's school systems at this time. As long as we're using speakers, films, and curriculum aids to tell children about the dangers of cocaine, marijuana, and other recreational drugs, why don't we add discussions on anabolic-androgenic steroids, growth hormone, and other performance enhancing drugs to this campaign?

The tie-in seems natural to me. I don't think it would be a waste of time or money to have schoolchildren learn about the dangers of performance enhancing drugs in addition to sex education, social diseases, recreational drugs, and the other topics covered in their junior high school and high school health classes. After all, studies like the ones I described in chapter 2 have shown that many students, and not just athletes, are using various drugs for pure performance enhancement.

# CHANGE ATTITUDES

Is big better? Is it cool to be macho? Is cramming at the end of a course to pass an exam (which really doesn't measure knowledge) worth getting involved with "uppers": caffeine, ephedrine, amphetamines (speed), and, yes, cocaine? This is a societal problem, and that means the so-called War on Drugs will never be won until the fighters turn their guns on the *need* for drugs.

We also need to recognize better professional and collegiate role models. Do we really want kids looking up to The Boz? Until the NFL and college football programs control anabolic-androgenic steroid use, until the game is returned to reasonably sized players, until the fans learn to appreciate a faster game requiring less strength and more speed and agility, bigness in sport will continue to be the rule. If you have to weigh 280 to 300 pounds to be a college lineman, forget it: We'll never stop AAS use in football.

I fear, however, until medical science can factually show that these athletes are suffering more injuries and shortened careers because of the drugs, we'll never get the attention of coaches and management. That brings us back to the need for research. Until AAS becomes a pocketbook problem for college sport and professional sport, we will have to wait for results.

## INITIATE EFFECTIVE, PRACTICAL TESTING

Say these drugs *do* become Category II controlled substances. Say we *do* spend more money on research and education. We all know that won't necessarily stop athletes from using performance enhancing drugs altogether. Human nature being what it is, we will continue to need drug testing—better and more effective drug testing!

It's obvious to me, after working with athletes for years, that the only way to ensure a level playing field is through dope testing. History suggests that for dope testing to be effective, the sports community is going to have to devise a new testing system, one that is scientifically accurate, fair to all competitors, and immune to politics and corruption. That's really all the athletes want.

What would be the ideal drug testing solution? How can we assure that all athletes, from all nations, are drug free? These are the million-dollar questions these days, mainly because, despite our best efforts, the international doping-control community hasn't yet come up with any effective solutions. We don't have a blueprint to work from.

However, I believe there are certainly options to explore, and I have some ideas that might go a long way toward clearing up the mess we're dealing with today. In fact, we may find that the solution to this problem is simpler than everyone thinks.

## INVOLVE THE RIGHT PEOPLE

We have already educated enough doping-control authorities, and we have learned as much as we can from this group. It's time we enlist athletes in the effort; we need their suggestions as to how they feel drug testing would be more effective. There is a huge counterculture in the AAS world out there that could be utilized. Former weight lifters, body-builders, and NFL players working together as a collective think tank could probably give us all we need to develop a nonbeatable test in several days' time.

Deep inside, I know from working with athletes (many of whom were drug users) that doing drugs was just part of doing whatever it takes to win. For many, sport was all they could really do. If they couldn't succeed in what they did best, the cause they had committed their lives to, because some other person was using drugs to get an edge on them, what was left in life? I know that even the athletes who have used drugs would have liked nothing more than a drug-free environment to compete in. When nobody could guarantee that, though, when the playing field wasn't level, they had no choice but to try to keep themselves even with the rest.

Now, however, those same athletes have begun to realize the detrimental side effects of the substances they once used. I bet we would all be amazed at the cooperation and knowledge athletes like Ben Johnson, Diane Williams, and Cindy Olavarri would offer if they knew they could help create a fair environment for future athletes, an environment where the next generation wouldn't be forced to make the same decisions they did.

Sport officials should offer clemency and anonymity to any athlete who would be willing to step forward and help us with his or her own information regarding how to beat the system or how to use drugs and get away with it. But, after seeing how Ben Johnson and others who were caught have been hung on stakes, do you really wonder why the silence persists? It is one thing to take medals away from an athlete caught red-handed, but I do not support the notion of stripping athletes of past records and medals, especially in light of the fact that we can't gauge to what degree doping has influenced all major competitions in recent years.

Another group I think should be included in some way with the development of a tamperproof drug testing system for sport is the media. Why not? They're watchdogs by nature. Also, I've grown to understand that members of the media often have as much insight and knowledge on a given issue as anyone.

Put it this way. In the 1980s, I've heard, most of the feature stories printed on baseball had to do with substance abuse. Not Pete Rose, not gambling—drugs. So, believe me, the media has been around the block a few times with regard to this issue.

I happen to think that the Olympic Teams of the United States are the property of the people, not of the USOC or the various NGBs. Therefore, we have a responsibility to be completely open and honest to the media, which links the Olympic Team to the general public. I suggest we not only open up more to the media but include the media more in an overall Olympic effort to rid sport of drugs.

## CHANGE AUTHORITY

In my personal opinion, if we're going to formulate an effective antidoping system, we need to move the responsibility for drug testing and education of the athletes away from the sport federations, which currently control this process, and establish an independent doping control agency. By giving supreme responsibility for the drug testing process to an entirely independent agency, we would be able to avoid that whole "fox guarding the henhouse" problem. History has suggested to me that allowing the sport federations to oversee even the best doping control processes has not been effective.

Let's set up an independent agency to assume *all* responsibility for doping control in the United States. If that means having the federal government step in and legislate a "drug act" to delegate all authority on this front to an independent agency, so be it. The sport NGBs and the USOC just shouldn't be forced to police themselves. For that matter, the NCAA, the national high school athletic associations, and the professional sports leagues shouldn't either.

On the international level, also, doping control for sport should be handled entirely by an independent regulatory agency. How would an agency like this be funded? Aside from corporate involvement, I believe all sport federations worldwide should be mandated to proportionately fund the international doping agency. This operating budget could be determined by the IOC and the agency itself. If a national delegation doesn't contribute, the nation doesn't compete. It's just that simple. In addition, each nation's independent drug agency would be subject to review by the international agency. Thus, all policy and procedural guidelines would remain uniform around the world.

This seems to make sense. The only limiting factors here would be IOC, international federation, and national Olympic committee egos.

## IMPLEMENT THE PLAN

How should the testing be done? What kind of nuts-and-bolts procedures should be followed to crack down on drug use in sport? Too often, drug testing officials try to lump the various forms of doping together in one science, and that can be a wasteful mistake. Because athletes are using so many different drugs in so many ways, I will approach each class of doping violations as a separate entity.

## Stimulants, Beta-Blockers, Narcotics, and Diuretics

Despite their different functions, these drugs all share one thing in common: They are taken around the immediate time of the athlete's event. Their use can be seen in any urine test taken 0 to 48 hours after use or after the event. Doping control for these drugs is therefore relatively easy.

I believe after-competition testing, the kind used while I was with the USOC, does a satisfactory job of controlling this problem. It's just the ticket. I wouldn't underplay the importance of after-competition testing.

As I have explained, athletes can only benefit from stimulants and other drugs in this category if these drugs are taken immediately before a given competition. For example, if an athlete wanted to use ephedrine to help him get hyped for a race or use beta-blockers to help him shoot better, he would need to take his particular drug just minutes to hours before his event. Metabolites of these substances can then be found in the urine up to 48 hours, or even longer, after the athlete had stopped taking them.

With particular regard to stimulants, however, there is presently a major loophole in the American testing system. In the case of IOC drug testing, any amount of banned substance found in an athlete's urine sample is considered positive. The USOC, on the other hand, chooses to address the situation of so-called inadvertent or innocent use of these drugs. If, on appeal of a positive test, the athlete can make a believable excuse that the substance was taken by mistake, such as is the case with many over-the-counter cough and cold medications, the USOC will let him or her off the hook on a one-time-only basis.

This is probably fair to the inadvertent user, but it does not protect other competitors from having to compete against someone whose performance is chemically enhanced. It is impossible to say the stimulant-using athlete does not compete with an unfair advantage. Any amount of drug in the system counts for some stimulant effect, at least theoretically. Unfortunately, this is another area that needs research to be cleared up.

If, however, inadvertent or innocent use can be documented, certainly the athlete should be exonerated. The competition, on the other hand, should be invalidated and replayed. This would be only fair to those who lost and tested negative: They would be given a second, fair chance. It would also remove the stigma that the innocent winner was or is a cheater. This being the case, more responsibility would be placed on the shoulders of the individual athlete in terms of what he or she takes before or during competition.

## Anabolic-Androgenic Steroids

Why are the tests for AAS now considered beatable by the athlete culture? The reason is athletes can use these drugs during training but stop using them in time to clear all metabolites out of their systems. The problem doping control authorities face here is *timing*. Any athlete with a brain and a calendar can use anabolic-androgenic steroids to benefit today with little or no fear of detection.

I believe there are several ways around this problem. If we are going to catch athletes who use anabolic-androgenic steroids, we will have to catch them when they're using the drugs: when they're training. One way to do this is by random, unannounced testing. In other words, track down the athletes who need to be tested, at any time of the day or night, and demand that they produce a urine sample for analysis. Doping control wouldn't tell them when they were coming; a knock on the door would be their only advance warning that they would be drug tested. By that time, if the athletes were indeed on the juice, there would be nothing they could do about it. How about that for action?

Some countries already have this type of program. The Scandinavians—the Swedes and Norwegians in particular—do such unannounced testing. Believe me, it works, at least when they are able to surprise the athlete. That is very difficult to do, though, because the testing officials seldom are able to make all of the planned athlete contacts.

I really can't envision a program like this working in the United States. First of all, a program like this would never withstand the pressure of organizations such as the American Civil Liberties Union and various players unions—with good reason. This SWAT-team approach to drug testing would be a gross violation of individual rights. I just can't justify dragging athletes out of their beds in the middle of the night to ask them to urinate in a bottle. This is not only degrading but also a violation of the U.S. Constitution.

Imagine also, if you will, the enormous expense of trying to track down an athlete who might be in Rome one week, Tokyo the next, and New York the next week, all in an attempt to run one urinalysis test. You can understand why such a system wouldn't work; doping control agencies would exhaust their entire budgets going after only several dozen athletes.

Also, the communication network of athletes is extraordinary. For example, I once tested Swedish athletes at American universities. Sometimes, the minute the drug crew hit the campus front gates, athletes were already in the next county. It proved to be a tremendous financial burden trying to pin down athletes targeted for testing.

The USOC and various NGBs have implemented a variation of this type of program, that is, short-notice (24- to 48-hour), random out-of-competition testing. I should first admit that while I was with the USOC, I essentially suggested that the short-notice approach be used. I felt by at least granting short notice, the USOC could avoid the search-and-seizure nature of testing programs like the Scandinavians'.

In having time to rethink this situation, however, I no longer believe in the concept of random testing. My reasoning is as follows: If we were to give athletes a 24- to 48-hour notice of testing, and *if* the notification process could be kept strictly confidential (this is a very big "if"), in practice this system might work. Based on the fact that the testing authority gives some advance notice of testing procedures to the athlete, this system just might withstand legal challenges.

This system, however, like unannounced testing, would ultimately be doomed to failure under the incredible weight of inherent logistical and financial problems. Such testing could become so expensive that it could destroy sport completely. Also, any system that depends on the concept of random testing could still allow the sophisticated user, once tested, time to bulk up before a key competition.

My personal prediction is that continuation of this type of program (the same program being designed for the USSR-USOC drug testing agreement) will ultimately prove to be an ineffective endeavor and an unfortunate waste of time and money. Random out-of-competition testing leaves too much opportunity for manipulation of the system. I have heard from athletes that they already have sources within the testing system who are willing to tell them exactly when the drug testing will be and who will be tested. If this is true, then any random testing program would be rendered completely ineffective. All it takes is one leak in the system, and the program fails.

The sad thing about random testing is that although every athlete is technically eligible to be tested, many will not actually be tested. Though the threat of being tested may or may not be enough to deter some users, I don't think it is enough to dissuade the athlete who chooses to use drugs only because he's afraid his competition is getting an edge on him. This was why sink testing failed.

Amateur sport has to have a system that can put every drug-using athlete at risk and can convince all athletes they will be tested. Any system that threatens to test only a handful of athletes chosen on a random basis won't work because the athletes won't trust it. If athletes don't trust the system, if they believe their competitors are still able to use drugs and gain an edge, they, too, will do anything in their power to beat that system.

Therefore, something better than short-notice, random out-of-competition testing needs to be devised.

### The Issue of Biochemical Profiling

Many other professional minds are already beginning to forecast failure for short-notice, random out-of-competition testing. That is why we are beginning to hear from such experts as Professor Manfred Donike, the "father" of modern drug testing, that a profiling system should be considered for what seems to be, thus far, an imperfect testing solution.

Profiling entails establishing an athlete's normal hormonal pattern on a urinalysis analytical screen. I'm told by scientists that such a profile is tantamount to a fingerprint because each person possesses a unique hormonal complement. This profile supposedly remains constant unless the individual's hormonal balance is tampered with. That is to say if an athlete takes a hormone (remember that AAS are indeed hormones) it will upset this picture and suggest that foreign hormones have been used by the athlete in question.

In order for profiling to work, however, certain hurdles must be crossed. The testing laboratory will need multiple tests that could collectively track any given athlete's profile over the course of months to years. Also, tests an athlete had taken years ago to establish his or her profile will be used against the individual by doping authorities forever. Once again, we find the question of whether such practices violate constitutional rights. Would United States courts allow past evidence to be used against a defendant a second, third, or fourth time? Heck no. In this regard, I'm afraid a drug testing system built on the practice of profiling may again take the concept of search and seizure too far.

Another legal conern I have about profiling is that the profile test does not actually identify chemical substances in an athlete's urine sample. Basically, the profiling system relies completely on circumstantial evidence. Rather than singling out drug metabolites, a profile test identifies the levels of various natural hormones in the body. A variance in natural hormone levels would significantly alter a person's biochemical fingerprint. If this profile changes, the testing agent will know something is amiss, though having no direct evidence of what substance had been taken.

Now, this can be a two-edged sword. First of all, a small amount or a brief cycle of anabolic-androgenic steroids may not upset a person's hormonal balance enough to alter the profile. On the other hand, prolonged use of AAS can significantly, consistently, upset the balance: The original, reference profile may be made by a drug user; he or she could then use drugs freely for years if the profile didn't vary from that first profile. It's unlikely, though, that the athlete would stick to taking the same dose for an extended period.

Therefore, the profiling system might detect only past use of AAS. An athlete could then argue that the positive profile test does not represent doping relative to the competition at hand, so profiling cannot be used as a complete drug testing system. Moreover, with new, synthesized hormones, an athlete could tailor an abnormal profile to look normal. No system will ever be immune to the threat of process manipulation.

On the other hand, a profiling system could be useful to doping control authorities because it may easily expose patterns of continuous past drug use by athletes. This would assist indirectly in determining if an athlete had been accidentally exposed to AAS.

For example, the precedent for such use of profiling technology was set by the IOC Medical Commission at the 1988 Olympic Games in Seoul. Doctors were able to use Ben Johnson's profile to determine that he had indeed been using anabolic-androgenic steroids for an extended period before the Games and that his water bottle had not been spiked with stanozolol, as he had initially claimed.

## THE BEST SOLUTION

For the immediate future, we need to find a more practical, reliable, and financially reasonable way to use drug testing as a means against doping in sport.

After-competition testing is a time-proven deterrent to use of stimulants, beta-blockers, diuretics, and other drugs used by athletes just before or during competitions. This type of testing is accepted and working, not only in the sports world but in societal programs in general. It must therefore not be deemphasized. We need to build from this system.

What is missing here is a way to prevent athletes from bulking up with AAS before competition and stopping use of these drugs in time to escape detection at a given event. If we can control drug use during the precompetition phase of training, I believe we can master the solution. If, however, we think some program of random out-of-competition testing on a year-round basis could ever conceivably stop AAS use during precompetition periods, we are probably mistaken, for reasons I have already detailed.

We *can* develop a testing program that could clean up AAS use among athletes just prior to and during competitions. This would guarantee for the athletes the most level field of play sport officials worldwide could provide. I suggest that the following drug testing program be developed by any sport organization that is serious about countering drug abuse among athletes.

1. Maintain after-competition testing at all major state, national, and international meets. Test all sports. Test for all drugs used to enhance physical performance in each particular sport. Seek support for continuation of after-competition dope testing by the NCAA in all sports at the conference and national level. Encourage professional sport organizations to do after-competition testing. Ultimately establish testing programs at the high school level.
2. To control AAS use, a precompetition test should be developed as follows. Sport administrators should require at least a 12-week registration deadline before *all* major competitions. Those athletes registered to compete should be informed and then subjected to short-notice (48- to 72-hour) drug tests at any time within that

12-week period, beginning with a test at registration. It should also be understood that any registered athlete *could* be tested multiple times within the 12-week period. For all major events, such as the Olympic Trials, all athletes would be tested at least twice. This would essentially shut down all the major precompetition advantages that could be gained through AAS use. Such times are when these drugs are most effective, but they are also when the drugs can be effectively controlled.

With this type of a program, athletes would have to seriously consider stopping use of AAS even weeks in advance of the 12-week registration cutoff. I understand from athletes most AAS take 3 to 4 weeks to clear the body. Thus, a user would have to be AAS-clean 15 to 16 weeks before the competition.

At that point, use of these drugs would be completely impractical. Over the course of 15 to 16 weeks, most if not all advantages that can be gained through anabolic-androgenic steroids would disappear. Even if athletes were tested at the 12-week mark and they wanted to gamble that they would not be tested again during the precompetition period, there would only be a 6- or 7-week window of opportunity for them to cycle again. And short cycles have been shown to be relatively ineffective.

Consider the hypothetical case of AAS-using Athlete Q. To prepare for national competitions, Athlete Q cycles down with stanozolol, taking only this substance during that last 3 or 4 weeks of his AAS cycle and then staying AAS-free during the 3 weeks immediately preceding a meet. Athlete Q has never failed an after-competition drug test.

Now there comes a new doping control system: Athlete Q is confronted with the possibility of being tested any time after he registers to compete in the U.S. Nationals. He wants to compete at Nationals—that's the premier event of the year. Once he signs up, however, he knows he will be called at some point and told that he has 2 days to report to a local doping control station to give a urine sample, or that a drug crew will visit him after practice in 48 hours, or something like this. He might be called at the 12-week mark, and maybe not again until the 6-week mark, but he *will* be called twice.

If he's smart, he'll decide to clean up his act before he even registers for the event. That means for approximately 15 weeks before his competition, Athlete Q will be drug free. Thus, most of the advantages derived through AAS use will have dissipated by the time be competes. In 12 weeks, even the aggressiveness associated with roid rage disappears. For that reason Athlete Q will soon realize there is no advantage to AAS use whatsoever.

For the sake of argument, however, say this isn't a major competition and there's only one required drug test. Athlete Q passes a drug test at Week 10 but then decides he wants to take the gamble that he won't be tested again before the competition. Even if he guesses right and is not tested during the remaining weeks before his competition, he will still have to prepare for the after-event testing. That means he can use AAS only between the 9th and 3rd weeks before the competition if he wants to leave himself a safe 3 to 4 weeks to clear his system of stanozolol metabolites. In this case, he's really pressing his limits; the odds may even be against his clearing certain after-competition drug tests. Besides, a 6-week cycle isn't that effective anyway.

Testing officials don't have to violate anyone's individual rights with this system. No search and seizure, just part of the rules, baby: Either play or don't play. Signing up means the athlete agrees to take dope tests at any time between registration and competition.

When one thinks how most athletes compete in a few major events per year, meaning under these guidelines they may be tested four to six times over the course of the year, one realizes how the potential of getting away with AAS use shrinks. Of course, this might not stop the incorrigible user from only competing once or twice a year so that he or she has time to bulk up. In most cases, though, infrequent competition may just counteract any advantages gained from AAS. Besides, an athlete can't compete in nationals without qualifying in previous competitions.

This type of testing is easy. The drug testing crew would know who will be competing. Officials would know athletes will cooperate because if they don't, they would be disqualified from the event. In this case, the athletes would have to explain to the media, their teammates, and their families why they aren't competing in the big event.

The testing agency in this situation would have a relatively simple job. Once registered, athletes are easy to keep track of, and they can be tested at any place, at any time, in accordance with policy guidelines presented to them before registration and with the logistical boundaries defined by the testing organization.

The issue of notice is no problem. In fact, the athlete would actually be given two notices: one in the terms of registration and one days before the actual precompetition test. In essence, this gives the athlete notice that he may be given notice that he will be tested! Now, who could ask for a fairer warning than that? An athlete could be tested more than once over the course of the precompetition weeks, but still this wouldn't be a violation of individual rights.

The agency sponsoring the event would incur the cost of drug testing. That would put the burden of providing a level playing field back on the shoulders of the sporting event organizers. After all, that's where fiscal obligation belongs.

Why haven't any Americans been ''caught'' for drugs in the past two Olympic Games? The answer is simple. All athletes who qualified for a team were tested at the Olympic Trials. In addition, those who made the Team were then placed under the jurisdiction of USOC drug control rules.

That meant they were made well aware of the fact that from the point when they made the team through the Games, they could be subjected to additional dope testing at any time.

When one thinks about it, the program I've just described is closely related to what I am proposing. Our successes in assuring that our 1984 and 1988 Olympic Teams appeared drug free only goes to prove how well this concept could work.

### Testosterone

Testosterone poses an especially difficult problem, but this method of testing could help control it. One should recall that testosterone, the natural male hormone, is the substance that athletes first started using to build muscles, strength, and aggression over 3 decades ago. It was testosterone that Dr. John B. Ziegler first witnessed Soviet athletes using during the 1956 World Games in Moscow. Though many new forms or derivatives of testosterone have been produced since that time in the vain hope of eliminating many of its masculinizing effects, testosterone still remains one of the most popular anabolic-androgenic steroids.

One of the main reasons testosterone remains popular these days is because, as the naturally occurring male hormone and thus not a foreign substance, it is the most difficult drug to test for. Finding the substance and its metabolites in the urine is normal. Whether the subject is male or female, testosterone is present, although to a lesser degree in women. Only when testosterone and its free radical epitestosterone are found in a ratio at or above 6:1 does its presence constitute doping.

The testing I've outlined can work in the same manner for testosterone as it does for AAS, actually helping the scientific community solve this testosterone riddle. In the proposed precompetition and after-competition testing system, observing changes in this ratio between two or several tests could help testers decide whether ratios up to and including 6:1 indicate an individual who is merely a variant of normal or one who is indeed using testosterone and significantly altering the ratio.

For example, say we test an athlete 10 weeks before a given event and find this athlete to have a testosterone:epitestosterone ratio of 5:1. At the event the athlete is again tested, but this time he turns up 2:1 (or even 1:1). We'll know he was messing around with testosterone foreign to his body because testosterone stays at a consistent level unless one unnaturally adds or removes it.

If the athlete in question tests a second time at or near 5:1, however, we can then pursue other biological tests to determine whether this is a normal variant or the athlete is suffering from a serious health problem, such as a testicular tumor. Until adequate research is done on this subject, no one will know what levels are verifiably "abnormal." Today's drug testing policies regarding testosterone are based on estimates and guesses.

Now, I should interject here that I consider a testosterone:epitestosterone level of 6:1 abnormal, but some of my colleagues believe a 6:1 ratio is not out of the realm of possibility for a person not using testosterone. Regardless, doping control policies shouldn't be based on guesses. As it is, athletes are either being falsely accused or let off the hook. We just aren't sure.

The doping control community simply must research and determine once and for all a reliable cutoff ratio for testosterone:epitestosterone among athletes. The type of testing I have suggested can help the process.

### Growth Hormone, Blood Doping, and Erythropoietin

That leaves us with the problem of how to control growth hormone and blood doping, the two doping methods for which there are currently no tests available to the sports world.

Growth hormone presents a serious challenge because synthetic growth hormone is now easily available and chemically identical to the body's natural growth hormone. Hence, urinalysis does not identify any metabolites. The same will be true with the new synthetic hormone erythropoietin, which is rapidly replacing blood doping as a means of increasing red blood cell (RBC) mass.

One solution on the horizon is to break down the legal barriers to using blood as the test material rather than urine. We have already managed (to a degree) to do this with blood alcohol testing, but there remains resistance due to the fact that taking a blood sample is perceived as an invasive procedure. (But in my mind, collecting a urine sample is also pretty invasive, at least as far as privacy is concerned). In many cases, individuals can refuse such a test.

The reason blood samples could help drug testing overall is that with research, natural levels of GH and erythropoietin could be standardized; we already have reliable standards for RBC mass. With such standards, the indicators for doping would be quite simple. In the case of blood doping, the reason for measuring the level of RBCs (the hematocrit) is that an excess of the standard would indicate doping.

This would fall into our concept of precompetition testing very well. All competing athletes duly registered would agree to a blood test during the weeks before competing; this requirement would be for everyone. The athletes would also be tested after competition. Taking a blood sample is fairly simple and not expensive. Most people have had it done several times. It would measure the number of blood cells weeks before competition and after competition. An increase in the level of RBCs after competition, if greater than the precompetition RBC level by a certain percentage (say 10 to 15 percent), would certainly be abnormal and would indicate that the athlete had either undergone a transfusion of RBCs or had taken erythropoietin.

I think it's possible to design a protocol for accurate and efficient testing for growth hormone and blood doping if a healthy commitment to research is made and changes are put in place.

## COST

Now, let's take on the subject of cost, the chief rationalization for weak drug testing. With the proposed system of drug testing, we will need a great deal of research support, but no more or no less than any other system used thus far. The most important area of research needed in the future to complement this system will be in the area of increasing length of detection for the shorter acting anabolic-androgenic agents such as stanozolol, oxandrolone, and trenbolone.

In addition, we need to research ways to follow trends in the use of designer drugs—not only designer AAS but also certain designer stimulants. Remember, these costs are a given. These drugs will have to be reckoned with by any system used. If not, the gurus will have won the game, and at that point we can all kiss fair sport good-bye. It would just be good business to invest in drug control because without it the entire value of sport will be nil.

The main cost to the consumer is the high cost of the test itself. Because the law of supply and demand affects the doping control business, however, an increase in the use of drug testing (not only for sport but for society in general) should push the overall cost of lab analysis downward. This in turn will allow for more testing at different levels of competition. As the next few years go by, new analytical methods will likely be developed to provide less expensive and more efficient analyses. All in all, costs should decrease.

## PUNISHMENT

This brings us to the question often raised regarding punitive action, sanctions that should be rendered against someone caught doping. In the past, I had been of the opinion that sanctions should be draconian, severe.

However, in a meeting in Zurich, Switzerland, in the late 1980s, while a member of the subcommittee on doping for the General Assembly of International Federations (GAIF), I had a change of mind. At this meeting we attempted to find an answer to the issue of sanctions. The discussion was divided between those with my original line of reasoning and those with the line of thinking introduced by a representative of the International Weightlifting Federation.

This individual, also a medical doctor and experienced drug control expert, argued vehemently for the concept of *decreasing* the length of suspension for those who test positive for drug use. His point of view, based on his experience, was that the sanction should not be greater than 4 to 6 months because a weight lifter suspended for 2 years would simply drop out of the picture, use AAS without any concerns, train intensely, and then return after the suspension, having realized a tremendous strength advantage. It is therefore better to keep athletes in sport and controlled, to a degree, by shortening suspensions.

I now accept this point of view and feel in the majority of cases, a shorter suspension would probably be best. I now believe sanctions should be shorter and testing be more uniformly applied, at least for first-time offenders. In my opinion, the second-time loser, on the other hand, is an addicted cheater and someone who should be permanently disqualified.

I would even take the penalty system one step further once a trustworthy dope testing system were in place. I would like to see not only the athletes held accountable for their actions but also the various governing bodies, which are supposed to be fostering an atmosphere of fair play in sport, held accountable. We need to get tough with enablers—those who get athletes involved with drugs or help them beat drug tests. Coaches, trainers, officials, physicians, and others who become enablers should be banned for life from involvement in competitive sport. End of story.

Throughout this book, I've explained for you how certain governing bodies have not seemed completely interested in combating the drug problem for one simple reason: It's not good business. Drugs work. They can help athletes win gold medals. Gold medals attract public attention and admiration. Public interest and admiration of a sport and its competitors attract corporate sponsors. And corporate sponsorships mean big bucks, the very fuel that keeps the whole system running.

Why, then, would a smart businessman (and make no mistake about it: Amateur sports in the United States is *big* business) want to snuff out drugs, hampering medal production, which in turn could curtail public interest, which may ultimately take money from his pockets? He wouldn't, unless either the public is aware of the drug problem and demands that he clean up his sport (that seems to be the motivation of many born-again antidrug officials in sport today) or he realizes that drugs in his sport will ultimately cost him far more than a dip in medal production would.

What if we said that a national sport federation as a whole would be held accountable and penalized if it had a certain number of athletes caught for using drugs? I bet that would rattle enough cages to make doping control a priority item within each sport bureaucracy.

Say three athletes caught using drugs meant sanctions would be leveled against a federation. If the Bulgarian weight lifting team had three athletes test positive for drugs in international-event testing, challenge testing, or precompetition testing (testing done by independent authorities to avoid internal manipulation) at any point during a quadrennium leading up to an Olympic Games, the IOC disqualifies the Bulgarian weight lifting team from the Games. If three U.S. track stars were detected for drug use by any worldwide-event or precompetition testing, the United States couldn't send a track team to the Olympic Games.

Can you imagine the impact that would have? Believe me when I tell you that the absolute *worst* thing that could happen to a sport federation would be to be excluded from Olympic competition. The USOC is still suffering from the blow President Jimmy Carter dealt when he ordered a boycott of the 1980 Olympic Games in Moscow.

No gold medals. No sponsors. Bad business.

If an NGB executive director were faced with these potential penalties, we all could be damn sure he would do everything in his power to foster a drug-free environment in his sport. He would *have* to test all athletes consistently to be sure they wouldn't run afoul of the independent international tests.

The clean athletes would pressure for increased drug education and testing. Why would they want to pay for the cheating of others any longer?

Also, corporate sponsors who sink millions of dollars into sponsorships would demand that the various sports be drug free. The investment wouldn't be worth making if you couldn't be sure the team will be there when it counts: at the Olympic Games.

## COMMON SENSE

Sport officials should be trying to achieve simple, inexpensive, but constitutionally acceptable methods to test athletes.

Drug abuse in sport is just one manifestation of the whole pill-popping problem our society faces. Over the years, we have been brainwashed by television that every malady can be solved by a pill, a syrup, or an ointment. Thus, it doesn't surprise me that athletes would look at pills, syrups, and ointments as shortcuts to success. No one seems to understand that what really makes athletes successful are good genes, good coaching, good nutrition, and dedicated, intensive training. We're all responsible for the drug problem—physicians, coaches, trainers, and all others. What some officials are doing now is even making matters worse.

I recall the days when I used to give athletes shots of vitamin $B_{12}$. I shot up more butts and thighs! My philosophy was that $B_{12}$ was a placebo. It may have had some psychological impact with athletes but no miracle effects, and at least my $B_{12}$ shots weren't hurting anyone, right?

Today I'm not so sure. I may have been doing something for the athletes that wasn't going to physically hurt them, but it was suggesting to them that they needed something artificial, something other than hard work and a good diet, to succeed. This is an innocent mistake many sports physicians have made.

I think it's time to admit megavitamins aren't necessary for athletes; they do no good unless the user is vitamin deficient. Few Americans are vitamin deficient; no elite athlete is.

I think it's time to tell the truth about the bee pollens, ginsengs, guarnao, octacosanal, Gerovital, aloe vera, glandular substances, herbs, and so on. None of these products have ever been scientifically proven to benefit athletes. They're fakes. What's worse, they contribute to the attitude that athletes need to take pills, powders, and magical elixirs if they're going to be winners.

The USOC should bear more of the responsibility of education and promoting the scientific truth, that what makes good athletes are good genes, good coaching, good nutrition, and hard work!

I'm convinced that drug-free athletes and teams will eventually prevail, set the new records, win the championships, and so on. When we can accomplish this, a strong and forceful message will go down to aspiring young athletes, their parents, and the drug gurus that risking bodily harm isn't a necessary trade-off for success in sport.

This, the greatest message I can hope to convey, may prove to be the ultimate solution for getting drugs out of sport.

# 12

# The Big Picture

## *Building a Better Olympic System*

Aside from the drugs, aside from the cheating, there are many other serious problems destroying the U.S. Olympic movement. If we look at the big picture, I think we'll see that drug abuse among athletes is just one symptom of a more devastating underlying illness.

Why do athletes use drugs in the first place? They feel drugs help them be the best they can be. They think without drugs they can't compete with other athletes. Shouldn't that tell us something?

I believe athletes *can* succeed without drugs because I know some are winning without them today. World records *can* be broken without drugs. Drugs are *not* a necessary evil.

In fact, over time athletes will realize drugs are more debilitating than helpful. Remember, for every inch of muscle growth an anabolic-androgenic steroid user may gain, he also gains some of the negative side effects described throughout this book. For every 15-minute boost of energy a cocaine user feels, he experiences an hour of depression.

Drug use is a self-defeating proposition. It's like taking two steps forward and three steps back. Sooner or later, the athletes and their gurus are going to wake up and realize this.

But today, the magnetic appeal of drugs persists. Why? Because U.S. athletes aren't getting the resources they need to succeed from the only organizations with the authority to deliver them, the United States Olympic Committee and the International Olympic Committee. When our athletes aren't given the right resources to work with, they're going to turn to other options available to help them do whatever it takes to win. That's a fact of life.

Clearly, two things must happen if the USOC is ever going to sort through the mess it, in part, has created. First, someone is going to have to do a better job of running the business of developing and organizing our Olympic Teams. Someone—and I mean the USOC—is going to have to do more for the athlete and less for itself.

Second, the athletes need to be taught that drugs are unnecessary. That doesn't mean getting some high-profile doctor to travel around and lecture athletes on the dangers of drugs. It doesn't mean more newspaper articles, books, pamphlets, or brochures. Athletes know when someone is trying to fill them full of sunshine.

How will athletes be taught this lesson? Only when they see a verifiably clean athlete succeed. The day Susie Steroids goes out on the playing field and gets her butt kicked by Susie Clean will be the day drug use in sports goes out of style, but only when Susie Clean has absolute "proof" that she competed drug free.

If they were smart, the USOC and all sport national governing bodies would hope to see that day come as soon as possible, before the general public gets too disillusioned and sport goes down the drain altogether.

Someone has to build the ultimate athlete with superior technique, strength and conditioning training, workout patterns, understanding of diet and nutrition, and mastery of sports psychology—not with drugs. Someone has to create the next Ben Johnson and have proof to say he became the fastest man in the world on guts and talent alone. I think the USOC should want to be the organization to help someone accomplish this.

First it would have to start functioning more like a collective athlete resource center, as many of the people inside the U.S. Olympic Training Center have been trying to make it work for years. A smart resource center would initiate programs to interest and involve athletes from early ages. It would provide expert instruction and state-of-the-art training facilities to any promising athlete who wanted them. It would take care of athletes by offering them food, shelter, education, and health care. And it would develop athletes for a life after sport. It would reward them for their hard work and dedication, start to finish.

Many athletes turn to drugs to help them break into the elite level. Only when they become the elite are athletes able to receive the best training, coaching, and money. Young athletes must be nurtured to the elite level with coaching and training, not drugs. Someone has to put the horse back in front of the cart.

In my eyes the Soviets have become, in the last 30 years, our Olympic superiors—not because of drugs but because they support *all* of their athletes as they should be supported. In terms of athlete care and development, the U.S. still falls way short of the mark, especially where the American high school and collegiate sports programs do not have a hand in athlete development.

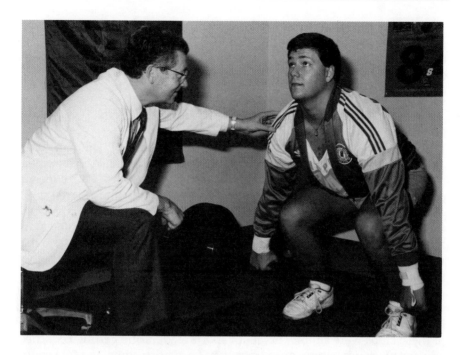

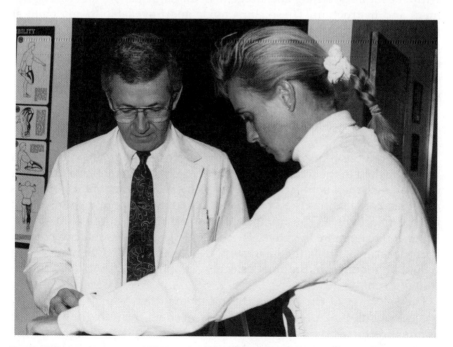

Part of the solution would be to initiate state-of-the-art programs, including providing facilities and education, to help athletes train to compete without drugs.

If we want to clean up our Olympic movement, then our programs, attitudes, and philosophies must change. Here are a few thoughts I've had, after working inside the five rings, that would help effect such changes.

## BUILD OLYMPIC SPORTS CLUBS

While with the USOC, Sports Science Director Charles J. Dillman, PhD, and I actively sought ways to improve the amateur athlete development and care process in the United States. The Olympic Sports Club concept, created by Dillman and Baaron Pittenger, is an idea that I agree with.

Many sports authorities have analyzed the Eastern European system for clues as to how they have selected and prepared athletes for international competition. The general conclusions by Americans are that we cannot copy their system because of societal differences and that we should base our own system on "the American way."

However, there are some features of the old East German system that can assist us in improving the American system. At the heart of the old East German athletic machine was the local sports club. The characteristics of these clubs were simple: excellent sports leaders and certified coaches, adequate facilities, strong encouragement for participation, and free equipment and instruction. These clubs made sport available to any child at no cost. By having well-trained coaches at this level, children received good introductions into sport, and the coaches themselves used this experience to select promising talent meriting further advancement in the system. If there was a "secret" to the East German success, it was these local sports clubs, which provided the base of operation for their system. If the United States can take a long-term view of building an effective amateur sports system, the concept of the local sports club should be developed.

To test out the concept of an Olympic Sports Club, a pilot study could be established in the following manner. Select a moderate-size city (over one-half million in population) that has demonstrated an interest in sports activities and also has the potential of obtaining corporate sponsorship for sports activities. The number of sports included in the club should be limited to no more than five. These should be activities that are popular in the local area, fitting the interests of the community. NGB involvement would be required in the final selection of sports to be included in this training center.

The selection of the staff is the most important aspect of this pilot project. A full-time professional staff is needed, including a high-level sports director who can promote and establish a quality program. Full-time, well-paid coaches for each of the sports are essential for the operation of the program. Other support staff will also be needed, including medical and scientific personnel to work with the coaches in establishing high-quality training programs. Perhaps these additional programs could be contracted with local groups if these capacities are available. The scientific group working with this club would then concentrate only on the sports included in the center. The NGBs could select the coaches, who would be paid a full-time salary by the USOC to work in the training center.

It would be ideal for the Olympic Sports Club to have its own facilities, but this may be impractical in some situations. Thus, some local facilities may have to be leased. However, it is important for the sports club to have its own identity, and some very visible facility would have to be rented or constructed to give the club a presence in the community.

The staff of the Olympic Sports Club would establish good working relationships with the community (coaches, recreational leaders, school teachers, etc.). They would run promotion programs on their sports for the community. With the assistance of the medical and scientific group, the staff would select and invite talented kids for trial participation in the Olympic program. Those athletes who seem to have the talent would be supported to train in their sports. These athletes would live at home, but once a day they would be provided transportation to the center and receive high-level coaching and training. All costs associated with training (coaching, transportation, equipment, etc.) would be covered by the club.

The basic purpose of the Olympic Sports Club would be to provide talent for the national program within a NGB. It is anticipated that the staff of the club would run sports programs for the local community and might even make the facilities available to the community as a fitness club during off-hours. In addition, the coaching staff should work with the local coaches as well as run educational programs that would have a significant effect upon the area's level of coaching.

How would we fund the Olympic Sports Club program? In socialist countries, the government pays for everything, but that's not necessary here. The United States is a capitalist country. The USOC already relies on the backbone of a capitalist nation, private industry, to help fuel the American Olympic machine. I believe corporate America could improve its relationship with the USOC, in terms of realizing greater value for its investment, and produce a better prepared Olympic Team. Concepts like the Olympic Sports Club could accomplish both objectives. First, however, the USOC must be willing to include this nation's best business minds in the overall program, and that means more than accepting checks.

## INVOLVE CORPORATE AMERICA EFFECTIVELY

If we want to be an Olympic power as a nation, I believe the corporations that sponsor the U.S. Olympic Team ought to be more involved with the decisions of where, when, and how the money gets spent.

I have always liked the idea of having corporations "adopt" a team. To me, that means more than a sponsorship: It's a partnership. For a corporation to adopt a team, it would take a given national team and provide not only funds but jobs, housing, and health, injury, and liability insurance to the athletes. The corporation could also offer certain career opportunities previously unavailable to many elite athletes in the United States.

The Olympic Job Opportunities Program is a bright spot in the USOC. In fact, I think this is one of the programs in the organization with the greatest impact. The USOC should expand this program 100 times.

There are ways to do this. Let's look, for example, at the sport of speed skating. Many of the American speed skaters train outside of Milwaukee. If a large Milwaukee company wanted to be an Olympic Team sponsor, it could adopt the speed skating team. The company would give the athletes internship-type jobs or educational opportunities. These programs would help the athletes prepare for life after sport. The adoptive parent company would allow the athletes time to train at the Olympic Sports Club. Perhaps the athletes could work or study 5 hours a day and train 5 hours a day.

In this system the sponsor gets much more than the right to use the Olympic rings on its product labels. The sponsor company gets to be more active in actually shaping the individual and the team. The sponsor sees where the money is spent and gets some sweat equity returned for its dollar, in addition to all the deserved public recognition. To top that off, employee pride would be a tremendous asset gained by the sponsor company. Successful corporations know what a necessity employee pride, loyalty, commitment, and support is to their overall operations. Imagine the emotions a company employee might feel while watching a co-worker, a young kid whom he or she's seen develop, earn a berth on the United States Olympic Team—and perhaps even win a medal! Now, that's something everyone would be proud of because they all shared in the quest.

I think people would be surprised what a little security, a promise of life after sport, and an environment conducive to individual success could do for an individual athlete as well as for a country's sports effort.

In general, I would like to see the training of U.S. athletes become more decentralized. Rather than a handful of Olympic Training Centers isolated throughout the country, I think we need to see numerous, smaller, yet multisport satellite facilities in the United States growing talented athletes and future business leaders—facilities like the Olympic Sports Clubs. The less we have to uproot an athlete from family and familiar surroundings, the better he or she will train. The better an athlete trains, the better he or she competes.

We need to reassign much of the central power away from the USOC and give more power to the athletes and to those footing the bill. The

USOC should become a simple distribution body for corporate funds, a collective bargainer, and an event coordinator.

## LIMIT SPONSORS

The greatest thing Peter Ueberroth did for the USOC as it prepared for the 1984 Olympic Games in Los Angeles, in my mind, was that he showed us, with the Los Angeles Olympic Organizing Committee (LAOOC), how a good Olympic business should be run. Basically, he cut the total number of Olympic sponsors down to a relatively small, manageable number. Rather than having many different sponsors pay a proportionately small fee, he enlisted a handful of leading companies and charged them what was needed to stage the best Games ever.

This was an effective move for a few important reasons. First, it allowed the Games organizers the opportunity to oversee all sponsor activities. Ueberroth's people didn't have to worry about babysitting 200 or 300 different companies that each wanted to handle its Olympic involvement in one of 200 or 300 different ways.

Second, when a company pays $50,000 for sponsorship rights, it can cut a check to the USOC out of petty cash and walk away—$50,000 really isn't a lot of money to big companies. I like to call this type of sponsorship a "good deed" sponsorship. A company donates $50,000 to the team, thinking it has done its good deed for the quadrennium, and then walks away, thinking the money was well spent, regardless of what the USOC actually delivers in return.

Now, ask a company to pay $10 or $15 million for a sponsorship, and suddenly the good deed turns into a marketing investment. Obviously, this is too much money to write off as a donation to the Olympic Team. When a company spends $10 or $15 million, if it is smart, it will be sure to implement the types of integrated public relations, advertising, and promotion campaigns that will make the sponsorship boost sales. That's just good business. The more a company promotes its Olympic involvement, the more it promotes the actual Olympic Games. That way, everyone wins.

Use an analogy to better understand this idea. A man wants to build a restaurant that will cost $500,000. Now, he could get 99 partners to pitch in $5,000 each, but if he's smart, he'll find 4 other partners to put up a $100,000 investment each. Why? It's easier to work with 4 people than 99. Also, 4 partners would be a lot more serious about making the restaurant a success because they have a lot more at stake than do the 99 partners who put up only $5,000.

In a sense, this is how Ueberroth organized things in 1984, and it worked. In my mind, the Olympic Games are the premier athletic showcase in the world. If a company wants to sponsor the Games, it should pay a price to do so. If the USOC made Olympic sponsorships a valued privilege that companies competed for, the whole program would benefit. The Olympic effort only suffers when more and more companies are able to buy sponsorship rights at a basement price, then ride the promotional wave through the quadrennium. Unfortunately, this is what is happening in the USOC today. At some point, the USOC got money-hungry and sold the magic of the Games to almost any company willing to ante up. The USOC is opening the sponsor floodgates once again, and it's ultimately going to be bad for business.

I know, after working with the USOC for several years, there are people whose sole function in that organization is to separate corporate leaders from their money. They bring the businessmen to Colorado Springs, pull out the flags and banners, bring in recognizable athletes, and roll the Olympic videos. They tell them how great the next group of athletes are and how many gold medals we're going to win, then, when the patriotic juices are really flowing, they tell their guests to sign on the dotted line.

To a degree, that's a necessary evil. The problem is, someone is going to have to draw the line sooner or later. I can't count how many times I had to turn down checks from megavitamin companies or quack sports medicine product producers because I didn't think the USOC should award sponsorships to companies based solely upon their willingness to write checks. Doesn't it matter if the company is reputable?

To attract funding and support from smart businesses, the USOC must uphold its standards and also be a smart business. Otherwise, it will find the best athletes, professionals, volunteers, and corporate sponsors walking away.

## REWARD PROGRESSIVE THINKING

That leads me to another very important point. When the USOC first started, it was a tiny business with a shoestring budget to operate on. Today the USOC has a budget of approximately $250 million.

Folks, that means this organization isn't a tiny business anymore—it's a corporation. Let's wake up and run it like one. The first step that should be taken for this to happen is that attitudes must change. One of the biggest problems I have with the USOC right now is its lack of innovative thought. It has no mission statement, no written goals, no drive, no character.

Word on the street is that most of the old USOC staff members in Colorado Springs can hardly wait until 1992 rolls around. Why? Because they can hardly wait to see how well their progressive athlete programs pay off? Because they're excited about how the next batch of young athletes will do in the upcoming Olympic Games in Albertville, France, and

Barcelona? No, they're excited because the new Training Center in San Diego will be built by 1992, and they can't wait to have the USOC pay to move them all down to the sunshine, where they can set up their retirement homes.

Is that the type of attitude that builds winning companies? Hardly. Winning companies are made by innovators, hard-chargers, decision makers, and risk takers, people who are not only smart enough to know what their consumers need but also gutsy enough to deliver.

There aren't enough hard-chargers or innovators in the USOC today. Most of them were pushed out of the organization by the executive officers, who didn't like having people buck the system from within.

The USOC lacks guts and innovation, but it didn't used to. The reason for this is simple. The Amateur Sports Act of 1978 essentially gave the USOC a monopoly in the business of Olympic sport. After the novelty of the original change wore off, the USOC realized it didn't *need* to be innovative. In the world of American Olympic sports, the USOC is king, love it or leave it. This is tragic, because what we are now seeing is that the Amateur Sports Act essentially abandoned the very principles of capitalist competition this country was built on when it gave the USOC supreme power, and it has failed.

Why is the Coca-Cola Company a strong company? Because if Coke doesn't keep moving forward, innovating, taking risks, and meeting the demands of the market, Pepsi is going to put it out of business. Why is 3M so successful at manufacturing and marketing so many different products? Because, as they are often described, they are masters of innovation.

Clearly, the USOC needs to become a more innovative operation. It's time to bring about that change, even if that means reassessing the Amateur Sports Act of 1978.

## PERMIT LESS VOLUNTEERISM

One other problem characteristic of the way the USOC is managed has to do with the distribution of power among volunteers and staff members. In general, I would say the volunteers have too much control of this organization and the staff members too little.

It makes no sense to have volunteers, who devote a small percentage of their workweeks to their USOC responsibilities, making all major policy decisions that affect the organization. It is equally ridiculous to ignore the input of the paid staff members with regard to U.S. Olympic policy direction. Unfortunately, this is how the USOC works.

The reason volunteers have such a high profile in the organization is because the IOC Charter says they have to. I believe, however, there is a subtle difference between being in a high-profile position and being in a powerful position.

Former USOC Executive Director F. Don Miller showed how important this differentiation could be. Col. Miller used to draw criticism from many who worked in Olympic House simply because he restricted our presence in the spotlight. Our roles at athletic events and the USOC House of Delegates meetings were strictly limited.

Though many felt this took some of the fun out of working with the USOC, I now understand how brilliant this strategy was. By limiting the staff to just doing their jobs, Col. Miller drew an invisible line of responsibilities between us and the volunteers, ceding the spotlight to the officers but delegating the nuts-and-bolts work to those he could hold responsible for it. Staff members were to attend volunteer-run policy-direction meetings only to take notes. We were the ones, though, who wrote the formal reports and recommendations, which the volunteers would in turn simply rubber-stamp. Who was really controlling the destiny of the USOC at that time? The staff, and the USOC was strong and effective because of it.

Today, however, that has all changed. The volunteers are clearly steering the course for the USOC as it sets off into the 1990s. Unfortunately, though intentions, I'm sure, are honorable, many of those individuals do not have the time, the training, or the insight to be at the wheel. What is even more bothersome is that being a volunteer seems to give justification to being incompetent. If I had failed at my job as director of Sports Medicine and Science, I would have been fired. Period. Why? I was a professional, a staff member, and I was expected to perform well: That's what I was getting paid for.

If a volunteer officer sticks his foot in his mouth at an international event, his job isn't in danger. Why? He's a volunteer donating his time out of the goodness of his heart, so we can't criticize him. That's inexcusable. The title *volunteer* shouldn't be a shield to hide behind.

The USOC can't effectively operate if volunteers are directing all the policy and making all the decisions. The USOC should find some way of making decision makers be more responsible and concerned with their work. Maybe that means shifting the decision-making power to those who are already inside the organization and are already concerned and responsible.

Don't get me wrong. We need volunteers. It is just that they should not be controlling the destiny of amateur sport.

## DUMP THE GOLD MEDAL MENTALITY

There's another attitude that needs to be changed to restore value to the Olympic Games once again. Americans are notorious for their gold medal mentality, as if gold medals were the only reason we send a team to the Games. We like to count the number of gold medals the United States wins, then compare that to how many the other countries win. We like to make heroes of the gold medalists and forget all the others. We have an attitude that first place is first but second place might as well be last. Go for the gold: That's all that matters.

I hate that. Maybe we're spoiled. Maybe we take things for granted. But I sure wish this would change.

What makes an Olympic hero? The amount of gold hanging from his or her neck? People who are really in the know about individual sports such as skiing, swimming, luge, and track and field realize that in many events, less than half a second can separate 10 or more competitors. Medal winners are often separated from the rest of the field by tenths of a second. Sometimes gold and silver medalists are separated by only hundredths, or even thousandths, of a second. Considering this fact, should we praise only the gold medal winners? I think all who compete at the elite level deserve praise and recognition.

Maybe we have something to learn from countries like Iceland, Taiwan, Peru, and Egypt, which rejoice as a nation when *one* of their kids makes it into the finals in *any* event, not to mention if, as luck would have it, the kid brings home *any* medal.

I sure wish the USOC, among others, would promote the Olympic Games as a celebration of the body human and a theater for international sportsmanship instead of some shopping market for gold medals or a place whose sole purpose is to have the Germans, Soviets, or Americans show how much "better" they are than everyone else.

Yet, the Steinbrenner Commission Report—that "earthshaking" document that was supposed to chart a clearer path for the USOC to follow in the future, but didn't—flatly states, "Winning medals must always be the primary goal."

I find this to be a narrow-minded, backward approach to nurturing Olympic athletes in the United States. I think the USOC needs to pay more attention to *how* medals are won than how *many* medals are won. If no one cares how medals are won, problems like drug abuse and politics begin to take control of sport. If the USOC were to pay more attention to the *means* to its end goal rather than the end goal alone, I think the medals would take care of themselves.

## *KEEP CLEAN RECORDS*

I believe there is yet another step we should take once we can ensure a drug-free atmosphere in international sport: We'll need to start a new record book. If we were able to effectively eliminate drugs from all competitions, at that point we should begin recognizing a completely new set of world and national records. There may be records on the books today that were set by drug users. Some records, though I believe they can be broken by clean athletes, may never be broken by an athlete without the aid of performance enhancing drugs, other experts feel.

Say, for example, we have a drug-free environment built for sport by the year 2000. If need be, we could then differentiate between all previous world records and all records set after the year 2000. I don't think we should toss out the old ones at all. We can't punish everyone for the crimes of a few. But we should *differentiate*, just because we can't be sure what was "real" and what wasn't. The old records don't have to be considered illegitimate or tainted, just "different."

Certain sports might just change the events. For example, so as not to degrade the 100-meter dash record, we could change it into a 110-meter event. The weight classes for certain sports such as weight lifting could easily be changed. The 90-kg class could become the 95-kg class. In this way we would not even imply that the old records were possibly tainted by drug use.

## A DOCTOR'S PRESCRIPTION

In summary, this is my prescription for making the USOC well again:

Most of all, we need to keep listening and learning. We all, like the athletes, have to keep striving toward our goal.

These ideas are just that: ideas! They make a nice starting point for concerned sports fans, coaches, parents, athletes, doctors, and trainers to go off and think up some of their own.

I have tried in my way to do my part, and I'm still trying. In medicine one must just identify or diagnose the problem; then the treatment is usually simple. I hope I have made several good diagnoses of the problems of elite sport, management, and drug abuse.

The treatments I have suggested must be reviewed, tried, and proven, but they may be the cure.

℞ For _u.s. Olympic Committee_  Date _____

Address _Colorado Springs, CO_

–Take better care of athletes. They deserve it.

–Decentralize the Training Centr concept. Spread the wealth.

–Get corporations involved in providing facilities and athlete care and development.

–Put realistic dollars behind the effort and manage the dollars well.

–Rely on professionals rather than volunteers for managing the USOC and sport federations.

–Start keeping real, drug-free records.

–Get off the gold medal kick. Medals will take care of themselves.

–Keep an open mind and be willing to learn, grow, and develop.

Do Not Write in This Space

☐ May substitute ☐ May not substitute

Repetatur _As often as needed_ Times

Do not label

DEA

Label

Dr. _Robert Cogg_

# Conclusion

Legend has it that Albert Einstein didn't speak when he was a young boy. This, understandably, was quite disturbing to his parents. Though he seemed to be a normal, healthy boy by all other means, the Einsteins couldn't figure out why little Albert wasn't talking.

So they took Albert to all sorts of specialists and doctors, trying to find a cure for his silence. In each case, the doctor would tell the Einsteins that little Albert was indeed normal and they should be patient: Nature would take her course.

Still, Albert didn't say boo.

Then, one night at the dinner table, a tiny voice finally peeped, "The soup is too hot."

Astounded, Mrs. Einstein asked Albert, "What did you say?"

He calmly replied, "The soup is too hot."

The Einsteins were overjoyed, but finally Mr. Einstein had to ask, "Albert, why didn't you say anything before tonight?"

And Albert said, "Because everything was fine until now."

Everything was fine until now.

I guess there will be critics who will ask a similar question of me: "Bob, if these problems have existed in amateur sport for some time, why did you wait so long to write this book?"

My answer would also be, "Because everything was fine until now," or at least it seemed that way.

Sure, I realized that amateur sport was tainted by drugs, politics, and money long before I ever got into this game, but I thought I could make things change. It took several long years to realize just how enormous and ugly these problems had grown. Once I finally realized the incredible depth of this situation, I also realized that I was not, after all, in a position to do anything about it.

Fortunately, word has gotten out to the public about drug use and politics in amateur sport, and for the most part, people don't like what they're hearing. The time is right for change. I hope this book has laid out enough facts to help people make those changes happen.

There is a quote attributed to the late Green Bay Packer Coach Vince Lombardi that goes, "Winning isn't everything; it's the only thing."

Another quote, this one attributed to Leo Durocher, then Brooklyn Dodger manager, goes, "Nice guys finish last."

Think about those quotes for a while. They're among the most popular, oft-used quotes in the sports world. "Winning isn't everything, it's the only thing." "Nice guys finish last."

What do they really say? To me, they indicate just how low we've stooped, just how far we've distanced ourselves from what sport really should be.

Let's face it. We're a sports society driven by an insatiable thirst for success. Everybody loves a winner, but nobody seems to care about how or why he or she won anymore. Isn't that pathetic? Is it really worth allowing a kid to risk life itself by using drugs, all in an attempt to bring home a shiny hunk of metal hung on a ribbon?

It's time we get back in touch with reality. It's time to care once again about the very principles sport is supposed to represent, principles like fairness, honor, and respect. Without these principles, sport isn't worth a damn.

Sure, let's cheer the winners, but let's cheer the individuals who win with grace, who win fairly, and who respect their competitors. For that matter, let's remember to honor all athletes who compete this way, win or lose. It really *shouldn't* matter if you win or lose, but how you play the game.

The day will come when the playing field is made level once again. I believe it, and so do the athletes. We have to believe that to be in this business.

I feel in my heart that these changes will happen. That's why I wrote this book.

If I can get one kid to throw away his drugs, if I can get to one potential user before she runs into a dealer, if I can convince one sport official to take a hard line on drugs, I will have won.

But the fight shouldn't stop there. If we want to stop athletes from doing whatever it takes to win, we ourselves must do whatever it takes to put the honor and fairness back in sport.

Get involved. Ask questions. Incite change. Demand fairness and honor, not gold medals. We all might be surprised what wonders the Olympic spirit can bring.

Otherwise, if the day ever does come when the sports world decides to turn its back on honor and fairness altogether, if we will have reached a point of no return with this "win at all costs" attitude, the gold medals won't shine as brightly, the flags won't wave as boldly, the torch will flicker dimly, and we will have lost one of the greatest treasures ever known.

# Endnotes

1. United States Olympic Committee. (1989). *Drug free.* Colorado Springs, CO: Author.

2. Burks, F.T. Drug use in athletics. *Federation Proceedings,* **40,** 2679-2680.

3. Dyment, P. (1984). *Annals of Pediatrics,* **13,** 602.

4. McLain, G. (1987, March 16). A bad trip. *Sports Illustrated,* cover, pp. 42-64.

5. Wadler, G.I., & Hainline, B. (1989). *Drugs and the athlete.* Philadelphia: F.A. Davis.

6. McLain, op. cit.

7. Goldman, B., Bush, P., & Klatz, R. (1984). *Death in the locker room: Steroids and sports.* South Bend, IN: Icarus Press.

8. Ibid.

9. Ibid, p. 24.

10. Ibid.

11. Staff. (1989, May 24). Ex-champion cyclist, herself a victim, warns about steroids. *NCAA News,* p. 26.

12. Prince George's County Court Judgment. (1986, April 21). *New York Times.*

13. Buckley, W.E., Yesalis, C.E., Friedl, K.E., Anderson, W.A., Streit, A.L., & Wright, J.E. (1988). Estimated prevalence of anabolic steroid use among male high school seniors. *Journal of the American Medical Association,* **260,** 3441-3445.

14. Scott, M., & Scott, M., Jr. (1989). HIV infection associated with injections of anabolic steroids [Letter to the editor]. *Journal of the American Medical Association,* **262,** 207-208.

15. Wadler & Hainline, op. cit.

16. Cooper, N. (1986, July 7). Cocaine is a loaded gun. *Newsweek*.

17. Gold, M.S. & Verebaj, K. (1984). The psychopharmacology of cocaine. *Psychiatric Annual*, **14**, 714-723.

18. National Institute of Drug Abuse. (1986). *Stimulants and cocaine*.

19. Harris, A.D., & Crawford, S.A.G.M. (1987, December). Drug abuse in sports. *New Zealand Journal of Sports Medicine*.

20. Harvey, R. (1989, May 9). IOC official questions drug testing in track. *Los Angeles Times*.

21. Litsky, F. (1990, June 14). TAC testing controversy brings about more charges. *New York Times*, p. D-24.

22. Harvey, op. cit.

23. Mirken, G., & Hoffman, M. (1978). *The sportsmedicine book*. Boston: Little, Brown.

24. Janofsky, M. (1989, April 4). Testimony on steroid use by Olympians. *New York Times*.

25. Woodward, S. (1989, April 4). Drug use alarming to Biden. *USA Today*.

26. Brewington, P. (1990, July 17). Controversial track coach banned for life. *USA Today*.

27. Woodward, S. (1989, April 6). Reputation led athletes to "steroid guru." *USA Today*.

28. Tod einer sportlerin. (1987, September 7). *Der Spiegel*, pp. 228-253.

29. Swift, E.M., & Sullivan, R. (1988, September 12). An Olympian quagmire. *Sports Illustrated*, pp. 38-42.

# Glossary

**acromegaly**—A condition caused by a surplus of GH in the body. Symptoms include enlargement of all connective tissue, as well as bone and soft tissue causing enlargement of the jaw, the forehead, the hands and feet, and internal organs.

**Amateur Sports Act of 1978**—Federal law that designated the U.S. Olympic Committee as the official national body responsible for amateur sports in the United States.

**amphetamine**—Stimulant used by athletes to increase heart rate and allay inhibitions before competition. This drug was particularly popular before cocaine garnered widespread attention in the 1970s.

**anabolic**—Refers to constructive metabolism, especially in muscle building.

**anabolic-androgenic steroids (AAS)**—Substances some athletes use to increase muscle mass, power, and speed. Anabolic-androgenic steroids, derivatives of the natural male hormone testosterone, come in pill and injectable forms. All are potentially dangerous to the user.

**androgenic**—Literally, "male-producing." An androgenic hormone produces masculine body changes.

**Beckett, Dr. Arnold**—London biochemist, research scientist, and expert on anabolic-androgenic steroids.

**beta-blockers**—Drugs used in legitimate medicine to lower blood pressure and slow the heart rate. Used as dope in sport to allay anxiety and steady nerves.

**blood doping, blood packing, or blood boosting**—Using an intravenous blood transfusion to increase the number of oxygen-carrying red blood cells in the body. An athlete could use donated blood or his or her own previously frozen blood.

**brake drugs**—Substances, usually hormonal, used to block sexual and physical maturation.

**Brooks, Dr. Raymond V.**—British biochemist and expert in laboratory technology used to detect drug metabolites in urine.

**Cassell, Ollan**—Executive director of TAC and vice president of the IAAF.

**Catlin, Dr. Donald**—Medical doctor, pharmacologist at UCLA, and director of the Paul Ziffren Olympic Drug Testing Laboratory.

**clean**—Refers to being untainted by drugs. A clean athlete is drug free.

**crack**—Crystalline, smokable cocaine; extremely potent and potentially deadly.

**Creutzfeldt-Jakob disease**—A fatal neurologic disorder caused by a latent virus that contaminates the pituitary gland and can be transmitted by the use of human growth hormone.

**cycle**—Period of time during which an athlete uses anabolic-androgenic steroids. While training and using AAS, the athlete is "cycling."

**Dardik, Dr. Irving**—Medical doctor and first chairman of the U.S. Olympic Sports Medicine Council.

**diuretics**—Drugs that by their various actions on the kidneys cause excessive water loss. Used in sport as dope to lose weight. Also used as a blocking agent to dilute urine and prevent detection of drugs in urine analysis.

**Donike, Prof. Manfred**—West German biochemist considered the father of and world expert on the technology of Olympic drug testing.

**dope**—Drug used in sport to enhance mental and physical performance. Also, drug used to alter mental or affective state.

**ergogenic**—Literally, "work-producing." In sport, this refers to a drug that stimulates, enhances, or produces work or performance.

**erythropoietin (EPO)**—A natural hormone capable of increasing the body's level of red blood cells. It can now be produced synthetically and used by athletes in place of blood doping.

**estrogen**—The body's natural female hormone, producing female body characteristics.

**growth hormone (GH)**—Human growth hormone (hGH) is naturally produced by the body to invoke maturation and physical development. Some athletes use hGH, extracted from the pituitary glands of cadavers, to increase their body mass. Today growth hormone can be created in the lab through a DNA replication process; this type is called synthetic GH.

**Hanley, Dr. Daniel**—Medical doctor and first U.S. Olympic Team doctor.

**Helmick, Robert**—President of the USOC and member of the Executive Board of the International Olympic Committee.

**hypertrophy**—An enlargement or increase in size. With muscle hypertrophy, muscle fibers enlarge but do not increase in number.

**immunoglobulin**—Protein in the body that produces or indicates immunity.

**International Amateur Athletic Federation (IAAF)**—The international governing body for track and field.

**International Olympic Committee (IOC)**—The governing body responsible for overseeing all Olympic affairs on the international level, including Games preparations, Olympic format, world records, event rules, and fund-raising.

**juice**—Injectable anabolic-androgenic steroids. An athlete using nandrolone, for instance, is juiced, or on the juice.

**Kerr, Dr. Robert B.**—Medical doctor from San Gabriel, California, and author of the book *The Practical Use of Anabolic Steroids With Athletes*.

**Ljungquist, Dr. Arne**—Swedish, vice president of the IAAF and chairman of the IAAF Medical Committee.

**Miller, Col. F. Don**—The first executive director of the U.S. Olympic Committee, serving from 1978 to 1985.

**Miller, Gen. George**—Former secretary general of the USOC and retired three-star general of the U.S. Air Force.

**narcotics**—Derivative drugs of the alkaloid opium, such as heroin, morphine, and codeine.

**Nebiolo, Primo**—Italian, president of the IAAF.

**Pittenger, Baaron**—Former executive director of the U.S. Olympic Committee.

**polypharmacy**—The use or abuse of multiple drugs.

**Pound, Richard**—Vice president of the International Olympic Committee and president of the Canadian Olympic Committee.

**roid rage**—A condition caused by anabolic-androgenic steroid use whose symptoms are uncontrolled aggressive and often psychotic behavior.

**speed**—Slang for amphetamine.

**stacking**—Using multiple drugs and varying doses to intensify their effects.

**steroids**—All hormones are biochemically steroids.

**stimulants**—Drugs that can increase an athlete's metabolism, heart rate, and sensitivity to external stimuli and can promote feelings of euphoria and invincibility, such as cocaine, amphetamine, and ephedrine.

**testosterone**—The body's natural male hormone, producing masculine body characteristics.

**The Athletics Congress (TAC)**—The U.S. governing body for track and field.

**United States Olympic Committee (USOC)**—The national organization responsible for overseeing the United States Olympic effort, designed by federal law to be responsible for amateur sports in the U.S.

**Ziegler, Dr. John B.**—American doctor considered the father of anabolic-androgenic steroids, he introduced Dianabol (methandrostenolone) to U.S. athletes in the 1950s.

# Index